全国高等医药院校药学类实验教材

中药分析实验

（第三版）

主　编　刘晓秋

副主编　原　忠

编　者　（以姓氏笔画为序）

干国平（湖北中医药大学）

牛丽颖（河北中医学院）

刘晓秋（沈阳药科大学）

齐　文（沈阳药科大学）

原　忠（沈阳药科大学）

麻秀萍（贵州中医药大学）

中国健康传媒集团

中国医药科技出版社

内 容 提 要

　　本书为"全国高等医药院校药学类实验教材"之一。全书分为两部分，第一部分为中药分析实验的基本知识，介绍了中药分析实验的基本要求及注意事项、供试品溶液的制备方法和步骤、中药分析方法等。第二部分为各类中药分析实验，共编写了 20 个实验，其中包括单项实验，如显微鉴别、理化鉴别、薄层色谱鉴别，以及有毒成分限量、重金属、注射剂有关物质检查、各类有效成分的含量测定方法等；综合性实验如二妙丸、大山楂丸、双黄连口服液等的质量分析；设计性实验如消渴丸等分析方法的设计等。书中每个制剂均选自《中国药典》，具有很好的适教性。附录部分收载了常用薄层色谱显色剂的配制和使用。为适应普通高等教育国际化的要求，编写了英文对照内容，便于学生在阅读外文资料、撰写英文论文时参考。

　　本书可供全国高等医药院校中药学、中药资源学与开发、中药制药专业使用，也可供成人教育本科和专升本、高等职业技术学校相关专业使用和参考。

图书在版编目（CIP）数据

中药分析实验/刘晓秋主编 . —3 版 . —北京：中国医药科技出版社，2019.3
全国高等医药院校药学类实验教材
ISBN 978 – 7 – 5214 – 0886 – 7

Ⅰ.①中… Ⅱ.①刘… Ⅲ.①中药材 – 药物分析 – 实验 – 医学院校 – 教材
Ⅳ.①R284. 1 – 33

中国版本图书馆 CIP 数据核字（2019）第 039893 号

美术编辑　陈君杞
版式设计　郭小平

出版　**中国健康传媒集团** | 中国医药科技出版社
地址　北京市海淀区文慧园北路甲 22 号
邮编　100082
电话　发行：010 – 62227427　邮购：010 – 62236938
网址　www. cmstp. com
规格　787 × 1092mm $^1/_{16}$
印张　8 $^1/_2$
字数　167 千字
初版　2006 年 3 月第 1 版
版次　2019 年 3 月第 3 版
印次　2019 年 3 月第 1 次印刷
印刷　北京市密东印刷有限公司
经销　全国各地新华书店
书号　ISBN 978 – 7 – 5214 – 0886 – 7
定价　**25. 00 元**

前　言

　　中药分析是中药学、中药资源学与开发、中药制药等各专业课程的重要组成部分，中药分析实验对巩固课程的理论知识，培养动手能力、独立分析和解决问题的能力具有重要意义。

　　全书分为两部分，中英双语对照。主要内容包括：第一部分为中药分析实验的基本知识，介绍了中药分析实验的基本要求及注意事项、供试品溶液的制备方法和步骤、供试品的分析方法等。第二部分为各类中药分析实验，共编写了20个实验，其中包括单项实验，如显微鉴别、理化鉴别、薄层色谱鉴别，有毒成分的限量、水分、溶剂残留量、重金属、注射剂有关物质检查等，以及各类有效成分的含量测定法，如分光光度法测定生物碱、气相色谱法测定冰片和高效液相色谱法测定银杏叶中多种黄酮类成分等；综合性实验如二妙丸、大山楂丸、双黄连口服液等的质量分析；设计性实验如消渴丸等分析方法的设计等。附录部分收载了常用薄层色谱显色剂的配制和使用。

　　本书在前2版基础上，突出以下几个特点：①体现安全、有效、可控、均一、稳定的理念。系统地论述了中药分析实验的基本知识、基本内容，由单项实验到综合性实验和设计性实验，体现了从鉴别、检查和含量测定三个方面对中药进行质量控制。②着力引导学生掌握中药分析的方法。本书力求使学生牢固树立中药制剂的质量观念，具备综合分析中药制剂质量的能力，注意引导学生掌握中药分析实验的特点、原则和方法。对每个实验的原理和依据进行了详细阐述。③推进先进评价方法的实施并具有实用性：本书编写了中药质量控制中先进的评价方法，如一测多评和指纹图谱等。

　　本书中的中药是从《中国药典》（2015年版）一部中精心选择的品种，并且经过预实验证明方法可行、重现性好、设计合理。

　　本书可供全国高等医药院校中药学、中药资源学与开发、中药制药专业使用，也可供成人教育本科和专升本、高等职业教育相关专业使用和参考。

　　本书编写得到了广东药科大学梁生旺教授的指导和审校，在此深表谢意。沈阳药科大学中药分析教研室研究生程喜乐、王欢、徐夏菁、王承峰在本书的编写中给予了帮助，在此一并表示衷心的感谢。

　　由于编者水平有限，书中难免有不妥之处，恳请读者谅解，并批评指正。

编　者

2018 年 11 月

目　录

第一部分　中药分析实验的基本知识

Part 1　Elementary Knowledge of Experiment for Analysis of Traditional Chinese Medicine

第二部分　各类中药分析实验

Part 2　Various Kinds of Experiment for Analysis of Traditional Chinese Medicine

第一部分　中药分析实验的基本知识

Part 1　Elementary Knowledge of Experiment for Analysis of Traditional Chinese Medicine

第一章　中药分析实验基本要求及注意事项

中药分析实验是中药分析课程的一个重要组成部分。用于加深对中药分析知识的理解；全面了解中药分析工作的性质和任务，培养严肃认真、实事求是的科学态度和工作作风。

实验课程要求学生熟练掌握各种分析方法和操作技术，培养独立开展中药分析工作的能力。正确掌握实验教材中各类代表性药物的分析方法。为确保实验教学质量，每个实验者应认真做到以下几点。

（1）实验前做好预习，明确实验的目的要求，熟悉原理和操作要点，估计实验中可能发生的问题及处理方法，有准备地接受教师的提问。

（2）严格按实验规程操作，细心观察实验现象。

（3）及时做好完整而确切的原始记录。要用钢笔或圆珠笔书写，字体端正。原始记录应直接记录于实验记录本上，不许记于纸条上或其他本子上。

（4）为防止试剂、药品污染，取用时应仔细观察标签，杜绝错盖瓶盖或不随手加盖的现象发生。当不慎发生试剂污染时，应及时报告任课教师。公用试剂、药品应在指定位置取用。此外，取出的试剂、药品不能再倒回原瓶。

（5）爱护仪器，小心使用，破损仪器应及时登记报损、补发。动用精密仪器，须经教师同意，用毕登记签名。

（6）实验时确保安全，时刻注意防火、防爆。发现事故苗头及时报告，不懂时不要擅自动手处理。

（7）爱护公物，节约水电、药品和试剂。可回收利用的废溶剂应回收至指定的容器中，不可任意弃去。腐蚀性残液应倒入废液缸中，切勿倒进水槽。

（8）实验完毕应认真清理实验台，仪器洗净后放回原处，擦净台面，经老师同意后，方可离开。值日生还应负责整理公用试剂台、打扫地面卫生、清除垃圾及废液缸中的污物，并检查水、电、门窗等安全事宜。

（9）认真总结实验结果，按指定格式填写实验报告，并按规定时间上交。

Chapter 1　Basic Requirements and Announcements of Experiment for Analysis of Traditional Chinese Medicine

Experimental of Analysis of Traditional Chinese Medicine is an important part of analysis of Traditional Chinese Medicine for deepening theory knowledge, fully understanding the property and task of the work, and developing serious, practical and realistic scientific attitude and work style.

The experimental course requests student to expertly grasp various analytical methods and operational technique. It also trains student to have the ability to carry out the work on Analysis of Traditional Chinese medicine independently, and to master the analytical method of each kind of representative medicine in the experimental book accurately. For better experimental teaching quantity, every experimenter should observe the terms seriously as follows:

1. Preview the experiment content seriously before carrying out an experiment. Make good understanding of the experimental purpose and requirement, be familiar with the principle, experimental procedures. Full consideration should be given to the precaution of accident and to the settlement of the accident happened in any case, prepare to answer the questions teacher should ask.

2. Perform the experiment strictly according to the experimental procedures, observe experiment phenomena carefully.

3. Record original experimental data directly in experimental record notebook in time completely and accurately. Write with fountain pen or ball – point pen. Forbid to record on note paper or other books.

4. To prevent reagents and drugs pollution, carefully observe the label of them before using. Eradicate the occurrence of covering a wrong bottle capping or without cover after use reagents. While the immodesty reagents pollution occurrence, be sure to report to teachers in time. The public reagents, drugs should be used at appointed place. In addition, reagent and drugs taken out must not be poured back to original bottle.

5. Take good care of equipment, use carefully, in case the instruments damaged, register and report to replacing in time. It must be obtained by teacher to use the precise instrument, and be sure to register the signature after usage.

6. Guarantee the safety during experiment. Pay attention to prevent from fire and explosion all the time. Any indication of trouble should be reported in time. Do not do any disposal if can not deal with correctly.

7. Take good care of public property, economize the electricity, water, drugs and reagents. Waste solvent which can be recovered should be poured into the appointed container. It can't be leaved arbitrarily. Causticity aqua should be poured into waste liquor cistern, abso-

lutely do not pour into the sink.

8. After the experiment, Tidy up the experiment bench, all the instruments used should be cleaned and put in order. With all above have been done and the tutor's permission students can leave the laboratory. Students on duty are in charge of the public agent bench, floor, cleaning the rubbish and the dirty in waste liquor cistern. Check the water, electricity, gas, door and windows finally.

9. Summary experimental result seriously. Fill in the experiment report according to appoint format, hand in report on schedule.

第二章　供试品溶液的制备

中药的成分复杂，需要经过提取、分离、净化制成供试品溶液，才能进行分析测定。一般根据被测成分的理化性质与干扰成分的特性及剂型的各异等选择提取分离的方法。同一成分在不同的剂型中采用的提取、分离、净化方法可能完全不同。

一、提取分离

按提取原理可分溶剂提取法、水蒸气蒸馏法、超临界流体萃取法和升华法。

（一）溶剂提取法

选用适当的溶剂将被测成分溶出的方法称为溶剂提取法。所选溶剂应价廉，使用安全，不能与被测成分发生化学反应。常用溶剂包括石油醚、三氯甲烷、乙酸乙酯、乙醚、丙酮、乙醇、甲醇、水等。苷的提取可选用极性较大的溶剂，而苷元的提取则选用极性小的溶剂；游离生物碱大多为亲脂性化合物，多用极性小的溶剂，而当与酸结合成盐后，具有较强的亲水性，应选用极性较强的溶剂。

常用方法为萃取法、冷浸法、回流提取法、连续回流提取法和超声提取法。

1. 萃取法　取液体供试品，精密量取，置水浴锅上蒸发至无醇味（酒剂或酊剂），移入分液漏斗中，用溶剂振摇提取，合并提取液，挥去溶剂，残渣用乙醇或甲醇溶解，作为供试品溶液。萃取的效率取决于所选用的溶剂，溶质在有机相和水相的分配比越大，萃取效果越好。

2. 冷浸法　取供试品粉碎，精密称取一定量，置具塞锥形瓶中，精密加入溶剂，浸泡2～24小时，滤过，取续滤液作为供试品溶液。本法适用于固体样品的提取，适宜热不稳定成分。影响浸提效果的因素有溶剂种类、性质和用量、样品的性质与颗粒直径、浸提的温度和时间等。

3. 回流提取法　取供试品，精密称定，精密加入提取溶剂，称定重量，连接冷凝器，加热至微沸，并保持微沸。放冷后，取下锥形瓶，密塞，再称定重量，用溶剂补足减失的重量，摇匀，滤过，取续滤液作为供试品溶液。本法主要用于固体制剂的提取，适宜对热稳定或非挥发性组分的提取。

4. 连续回流提取法　使用索氏提取器连续进行提取，操作简便，节省溶剂，提取效率高。适用于对热稳定物质的提取。

5. 超声提取法 精密称取供试品，精密加入提取溶剂，超声振荡提取一定时间，取出，称重，补足溶剂减失的重量，滤过，取续滤液作为供试品溶液。这种方法简便、快速、提取效率高。

（二）水蒸气蒸馏法

适用于能随水蒸气蒸馏而不被破坏的成分。挥发油、一些小分子的生物碱如麻黄碱、槟榔碱，某些酚类物质如丹皮酚等可用本法提取。

（三）超临界流体萃取法

超临界流体是指高于临界压力和临界温度时所形成的单一相态，如CO_2的临界温度为31℃，临界压力为7390kPa。它既不是气体，也不是液体，但它兼有气体和液体的某些性质，即兼有气体的低黏度，液体的高密度以及介于气、液之间较高的扩散系数等特征。萃取后在常压状态下溶剂立即变为气体而逸出，可提到纯净的样品。

（四）升华法

取金属片，置石棉网上，金属片上放一直径2cm、高约8mm的金属环。圈内放置适量药材粉末，圈上覆盖载玻片，在石棉网下用酒精灯缓缓加热，至粉末开始变焦，冷却。将载玻片置显微镜下观察或取升华物加试液观察反应。

二、净化方法

提取液大多还需作进一步的净化分离，除去干扰组分后才能进行测定。净化的原则是最大限度保留被测定成分而除去对测定有干扰的杂质。净化方法的选择主要依据被测定成分和杂质在理化性质上的差异，同时结合所采用的测定方法的要求而综合考虑。常用的净化方法有以下两种。

（一）液–液萃取法

同提取分离中的萃取步骤。

（二）色谱法

精密量取提取液，除掉溶剂，将残渣溶解，用适当的色谱柱如大孔吸附树脂、聚酰胺、十八烷基键合相硅胶等柱处理。以适宜的溶剂洗脱，收集一定量的洗脱液，蒸干。将残渣溶解，混合均匀。

三、制备步骤

（1）一步提取，补足减失的重量，取滤液。

取样品，粉碎，加入一定量的溶剂（50～100倍），采用适当的提取方法（回流、连续回流、超声等）提取20分钟至1小时，放冷，补足减失的重量，滤过，滤液作为供试品溶液。

（2）多步提取，合并滤液，稀释至一定体积。

取样品，粉碎，加入一定量的溶剂（10～20倍），采用适当的提取方法（回流、连续回流、超声等）提取20分钟至1小时，滤过，滤渣加溶剂再提取1～2次，滤过，合并滤液置量瓶中，加溶剂稀释至刻度，摇匀，作为供试品溶液。

Chapter 2　Preparation of Test Solution

The Constituents of Traditional Chinese medicines are complex, so test solution should be prepared by extraction, isolation and purification method before analysis. In general, the method chosen should comply with the physical and chemical property of the determined and interferential constituent, as well as diversity of dosage form of Traditional Chinese patent medicines. There are different extraction, separation and purification methods for same constituent in different dosage form.

1. Extraction and separation

According to principle, extract methods can be classified into solvent extraction, vapour distillation, supercritical fluid extraction and sublimation.

(1) Solvent extraction　Solvent extraction is summarized as extracting the constituent determined by using proper solvent. The solvent chosen should be cheap, safe and can not react with the constituent determined. The common solvents for extracting include petroleum ether, chloroform, ethyl acetate, ethyl ether, acetone, ethanol, methanol, water and so on. For example, the solvent of high polarity is chosen for the extraction of glycosides, while the solvent of low polarity is chosen for the extraction of aglycone. Most of free alkaloids are lipophilic compound which can be extracted with solvent of low polarity. When free alkaloids react with acid, hydrophilous substance, salt, was produced, which can be extracted with solvent of high polarity.

Common methods include extraction, cold maceration, reflux extraction, successive reflux extraction and ultrasonication.

Extraction method　To liquid test sample, measure accurately, evaporate it (alcohol or tincture) on a water bath until no ethanol smell is perceptible, transfer it into a separating funnel. Extract it with certain quantities of solvent, combine the solvent extracts and expel the solvent. Dissolve the residue in ethanol or methanol as the test solution. The efficiency of the extraction is up to the solvent selected. The higher distributive proportion the solute is between organic phase and water phase, the more efficiency it is.

Cold maceration method　Place powder of test sample, weigh accurately, in stopper conical flask, add solvent accurately, macerate for 2 – 24 hours, filter, take the successive filtrate as test solution. The method is appropriate to the extraction of solid samples which are unstable under heating. The factors that influence the efficiency of extraction contain sorts, property and volume of solvent, property of sample and diameter of grind, temperature and time of maceration, and so on.

Reflux method　To test sample, weigh accurately, add solvent accurately, weigh again, connect to reflux condenser tube, heat, maintain boiling gently, cool, take off the conical flask, stoppered well, weigh. Add solvent to restore its original weight, shake well, filter, and take the successive filtrate as test solution. The method is appropriate to the extraction of solid sample, which is stable under heating or does not contain volatile constituents.

Successive reflux method Successively extract with Soxhlet's extractor. This method is simple, saving and highly efficient, appropriate to the extraction of the substances which are stable under heating.

Ultrasonication method To test sample, weigh accurately, add solvent accurately, ultrasonicate for a moment, remove, weigh again. Add solvent to restore its original weight, shake well, filter, take the successive filtrate as the test solution. This method is simple, swift and efficient.

(2) Vapour distillation method The method is appropriate to the sample which is stable under heating and can be distilled with vapour, such as volatile oil, some alkaloids of small molecule (ephedrine, arecoline) and some phenolics e. g. paeonol can be extracted by this method.

(3) Supercritical fluid (SCF) extraction method SCF is a substance state which is formed above critical pressure and critical temperature. For example, the critical pressure of carbon dioxide is 7390kPa, and the critical temperature is 31℃. SCF is neither gas nor liquid, however, it owns the property of both of them, low viscosity of gas, high density of liquid and high diffusion coefficient between gas and liquid. After extracting, the SCF will convert at ambient pressure. Then the pure sample appears.

(4) Sublimate method Place a metallic slide on an asbestos plate with a metallic ring of about 2 cm in diameter and about 8 mm high on the slide. Place a thin layer of powdered drugs to be examined in the ring, covered with a glass slide, heat gently under the asbestos plate until the powder is charred then remove the glass slide and allow to cool. Examine the crystal form and colour of sublimate condensed on the slide under a microscope or carry out the appropriate chemical tests on the sublimate.

2. Purification method

Before determination, the extracting solution needs to be further purified to remove the impurity. The principle of purification is to retain the ingredients determined and to remove the ingredients interfered maximally. The purification method selected is on the ground of differences of chemical and physical property between the constituents determined and the constituents interfered and must bond with the determination method. The common purification methods contain liquid – liquid extraction method and chromatography.

(1) Liquid – Liquid extraction method The same as the procedure of above (description in extraction and separation).

(2) Chromatography Measure the solution, accurately, expel the solvent. Dissolve the residue and apply the solution to a column packed with macroporous, polyamide, octadecylsilane bonded silica gel. Elute with proper solvent, collect quantities of the eluate and evaporate to dryness. Dissolve the residue, mix well.

3. operating steps

（1）One – step extraction, replenish the lost weight, and use the successive filtrate.

Take the sample, pulverize into fine powder, add a certain amount of solvent (50 – 100 times), use the appropriate extraction method (reflux, continuous reflux, ultrasonic, etc.), extraction time 20min – 1h, replenish the lost weight, filter, use the successive filtrate as the test solution.

（2）A multi – step extraction, combine the filtrate, and dilute to constant volume.

Take the sample, pulverize into fine powder, add a certain amount of solvent (10 – 20 times), use the appropriate extraction method (reflux, continuous reflux, ultrasonic, etc.), extraction 20min – 1h, filter, dissolve the residue with proper solvent to extract 1 or 2 more times, filter, combine the filtrate, and dilute to constant volume, mix well, as the test solution.

第三章　供试品的分析方法

一、鉴别

鉴别是指检验中药真伪的方法，包括经验鉴别、显微鉴别、理化鉴别。经验鉴别是用传统的实践经验，显微鉴别是指用显微镜对中药的切片、粉末、解离组织或表面制片的显微特征进行鉴别。理化鉴别包括物理、化学、光谱、色谱等鉴别方法。

薄层色谱法在中药鉴别中应用最为广泛，具有专属性强、操作简便等优点，并具有分离和鉴别的双重作用，具有重现性、专属性，用对照品或对照药材作对照判断鉴别结果，确认中药的真伪。

二、检查

检查是指药品在加工、生产和贮藏过程中可能含有的需要控制的物质或其限度指标，是对中药的含水量、纯净程度、有害或有毒物质、浸出物进行限量或含量检查。

三、含量测定

含量测定是指用化学、物理或生物的方法，对中药含有的有效成分、指标成分或类别成分进行测定，以评价其内在质量的项目和方法。常用的如经典分析方法（容量法、重量法）、紫外 – 可见分光光度法、高效液相色谱法、气相色谱法等。

四、分析方法验证的基本内容

中药化学成分的测定方法因品种不同，凡是自行建立的新方法，均要进行方法学考察研究。一般考察项目如下。

（一）准确度

准确度系指用该方法测定的结果与真实值或参考值接近的程度，一般用回收率

（%）表示。准确度应在规定的范围内测试。

1. 含量测定方法的准确度 于已知被测成分含量的供试品中精密加入一定量的已知纯度的被测成分对照品，依法测定。用实测值与供试品中含有量之差，除以加入对照品量计算回收率。

$$回收率,\% = （C - A）/B × 100\%$$

式中，A ——供试品所含被测成分量；

B ——加入对照品量；

C ——实测值。

2. 数据要求 在规定范围内，取同一浓度的供试品，用 6 个测试结果进行评价；或设计 3 个不同浓度，每个浓度各分别制备 3 份供试品溶液进行测试，用 9 个测定结果进行评价，一般中间浓度加入量与所取供试品含量之比控制在 1∶1 左右。应报告供试品取样量、供试品中含有量、对照品加入量、测定结果和回收率（%）的相对标准偏差（RSD%）或可信限。

（二）精密度

精密度系指在规定的测试条件下，同一均匀供试品，经多次取样测定所得结果之间的接近程度。精密度一般用偏差、标准偏差或相对标准偏差表示。

精密度包含重复性、中间精密度和重现性。

在相同操作条件下，由同一分析人员在较短的间隔时间内测定所得的结果的精密度称为重复性；在同一个实验室，不同时间由不同分析人员用不同设备测定结果之间的精密度称为中间精密度；在不同实验室由不同分析人员测定结果之间的精密度称为重现性。

用于定量测定的分析方法均应考察方法的精密度。

1. 重复性 在规定范围内，取同一浓度的供试品，用 6 个测试结果进行评价；或设计 3 个不同浓度，每个浓度各分别制备 3 份供试品溶液进行测试，用 9 个测定结果进行评价。

2. 中间精密度 为考察随机变动因素对精密度的影响，应进行中间精密度试验。变动因素为不同日期、不同分析人员、不同设备等。

3. 重现性 当分析方法将被法定标准采用时，应进行重现性试验。例如建立药典分析方法时通过不同实验室的复核检验得出重现性结果。符合检验的目的、过程和重现性结果均应记载在起草说明中。

4. 数据要求 均应报告标准偏差、相对标准偏差或可信限。

（三）专属性

专属性系指在其他成分可能存在的条件下，采用的方法能正确测定出被测成分的特性。鉴别试验、限量检查、含量测定等方法均应考察其专属性。

1. 鉴别实验 应能与可能共存的物质或结构相似化合物区分。不含被测成分的供试品，以及结构相似或组分中的有关化合物，均不得干扰测定。显微鉴别、色谱及光谱鉴别等应附相应的代表性图像或图谱。

2. 含量测定和限量测定 以不含被测成分的供试品（除去含待测成分药材或不含

待测成分的模拟复方）试验说明方法的专属性。色谱法、光谱法等应附代表性图谱，并标明相关成分在图中的位置，色谱法中的分离度应符合要求。必要时可采用二极管阵列检测和质谱检测，进行峰纯度检查。

（四）检测限

检测限系指供试品中被测物能被检测出的最低量。确定检测限常用的方法如下。

1. 直观法 用一系列已知浓度的供试品进行分析，试验出能被准确、可靠地检测出的最低浓度或量。

2. 信噪比法 仅适用于能显示基线噪声的分析方法，即把已知低浓度供试品测出的信号与空白样品测出的信号进行比较，算出能被可靠地检测出的最低浓度或量。一般以信噪比 3:1 或 2:1 时相应浓度或注入仪器的量确定检测限。

3. 数据要求 应附测试图谱，说明测试过程和检测限结果。

（五）定量限

定量限系指供试品中被测成分能被定量测定的最低量，其测定结果应具一定的准确度和精密度。用于限定检查或定量测定的分析方法应确定定量限。

常用信照比法确定定量限。一般以信噪比 10:1 时相应浓度或注入仪器的量进行确定。

（六）线性

线性系指在设计的范围内，测试结果与供试品中被测物浓度直接成正比关系的程度。

应在规定的范围内测定线性关系。可用一贮备液经精密稀释，或分别精密称样，制备一系列供试品的方法进行测定，至少制备 5 个浓度的供试品。以测定的响应信号作为被测物浓度的函数作图，观测是否呈线性，再用最小二乘法进行线性回归。必要时，响应信号可经数学转换，再进行线性回归计算。

数据要求：应列出回归方程、相关系数和线性图。

（七）范围

范围系指能达到一定精密度、准确度和线性，测试方法适用的高低限浓度和量的区间。

范围应根据分析方法的具体应用和线性、准确度、精密度结果及要求确定。对于有毒的、具特殊功能或药理作用的成分，其范围应大于被限定含量的区间。

（八）耐用性

耐用性系指在测定条件有小的变动时，测定结果不受影响的承受程度，为使方法用于常规检验提供依据。开始研究分析方法时，就应考虑其耐用性。如果测试条件要求苛刻，则应在方法中写明。典型的变动因素有：被测溶液的稳定性，样品提取次数、时间等。液相色谱法中典型的变动因素有：流动相的组成比例或 pH，不同厂牌或不同批号的同类型色谱柱、柱温、流速及检测波长等。气相色谱法变动因素有：不同厂牌或不同批号的色谱柱、固定相、不同类型的载体、柱温、进样口和检测器温度等。薄层色谱变动因素有：不同厂牌的薄层板、点样方式及薄层展开时温度及相对湿度的变化等。

经实验，应说明小的变动能否通过设计的系统适用性实验以确保方法有效。

Chapter 3　Analysis Methods of Test Samples

1. Identification

Identification refers to the authenticity of Chinese medicine, including empirical identification, microscopic identification, physical and chemical identification. Microscopic identification is a method of identifying the microscopic characteristics of slices, powders, dissociated tissues or surface preparations of traditional Chinese medicine by microscopy. Physical and chemical identification includes identification methods such as physics, chemistry, spectroscopy and chromatography.

Thin – layer chromatography (TLC) is the most widely used in the identification of traditional Chinese medicine. It has the advantages of strong specificity, easy operation, and the dual functions of separation and identification. TLC can be used to determine true and false by chemical reference substance or reference crude herb.

2. Limit Test

Limit Test refers to the substances or their limit indicators that need to be controlled in the processing, production and storage of medicines. It is a limit or content inspection of the water content, purity, harmful or toxic substances, and extracts of traditional Chinese medicine.

3. Assay

Assay refers to the determination of the effective components, indicator components or a class of components contained in traditional Chinese medicine by chemical, physical or biological methods, in order to evaluate its internal quality items and methods.

Methods such as classical analysis (volume method, gravimetric method), ultraviolet – visible spectrophotometry, high performance liquid chromatography and gas chromatography are commonly used.

4. Verification of Analysis Methods

The determination method of chemical component of the traditional Chinese medicine complied with individual monograph is different. If the new method is set up by ourself, you must have a study of the analysis method. Common study items are as follows.

4.1 Accuracy

The accuracy of an analytical method is the closeness of test results obtained by that method to the true value or the reference value. Accuracy is often expressed as percent recovery and should be in the specified range.

(1) Accuracy of the method for content determination　An amount of the reference substance with known purity of analyte is precisely added into the sample being examined with known content of analyte to be examined, and test accordingly. The margin of the determined value and the amount of the analyte in the sample is divided by the amount of the added refer-

ence substance to calculated the recovery ratio.

$$Recovery, \% = (C - A) / B \times 100\%$$

In the above formula: A is the amount of the analyte in the sample being examined; B is the amount of the added reference substance; C is the determined value.

(2) Requirement for the data　In specified range, the accuracy should be evaluated using 6 testing results of the sample, or 3 different concentration levels of the solution are prepared and each concentration level is measured for 3 times, 9 testing results. Commonly, ratio of intermediate concentration of added amount and content of test is 1 : 1. Amount of sample and its content, amount of reference added, test result, the recovery percentage and RSD should be reported.

4.2 Precision

The precision of an analytical method is the degree of agreement among individual test results when the procedure is applied repeatedly to multiply sampling of a homogeneous sample. The precision of an analytical method is usually expressed as deviation, standard deviation or relative standard deviation.

Precision includes repeatability, intermediate – precision and reproducibility.

Repeatability is the precision obtained by the same analyst within a laboratory over a short period of time with the same equipment. Intermediate – precision is the precision obtained by different analysts within the same laboratory on different days with different equipment. Repeatability is the precision obtained by different analysts using the same analytical procedure.

Precision of the method should be considered when the content of active ingredients determined.

(1) Repeatability　In specified range, repeatability should be evaluated with 6 measurements results when the concentration level of the analyte at 100% or 3 different concentration levels of the solution are prepared and each concentration level is measured for 3 times, with 9 measurement results.

(2) Intermediate – precision　Scheme should be designed to inspect the effect of random variable factors on the precision. The variable factors include different dates, different analysts and different equipment.

(3) Reproducibility　Reproducibility should be done when an analytical method is adopted as the legal standard. For example, result of reproducibility should be obtained by different laboratory when pharmacopoeia method will be developed. The objective and process of the collaborative study and result of the reproducibility should be recorded in the description of draft file.

(4) Requirement for data　Standard deviation, relative standard deviationor confidential limit should be reported.

4.3 Specificity

The specificity of an analytical method is its ability to measure accurately and specifically the analyte in the presence of components that may be expected to be present. Specificity should be inspected when identification, impurity test and content determination will be done.

(1) Identification　The compound that may coexist or have close related structures should be distinguished from the active ingredient. The sample without the tested ingredient, compound should all offer negative response when microscopical, chromatograph and spectral identification are used, the representative graphs should be recorded.

(2) Assay and limit test　Sample which does not contain constituent tested is used in experiment. The representative graphs should be recorded for verifying specificity when chromatograph or other separation methods are used. The position of each component should be marked in the graph. The resolution of the chromatographic method should meet the requirements.

4.4 Limit of Detection

The limit of detection is the lowest concentration of the analyte in a sample that can be detected. The commonly used methods are as follows.

(1) Noninstrumental method　The limit of detection is generally determined by the analysis of samples with known concentration of analyte and by establishing the minimum level at which the analyte can be reliably detected.

(2) Signal – to – noise ratio method　The method for the instrumental method which can record the noise of the baseline, the minimum level at which the analyte can be reliably detected, can be established by comparing the test results from samples with known concentrations of analyte with those of blank samples. A signal – to – noise ratio of 2 : 1 or 3 : 1 is generally accepted.

(3) Requirement for data　The test graphs should be attached, the test process and the results should be declared.

4.5 Limit of Quantitation

Limit of quantitation is the lowest concentration of the analyte in the sample that can be determined with acceptable precision and accuracy under the stated experimental conditions. The limit of quantitation should be determined when the quantitative determination for impurities and degradation products are developed.

Signal – to – noise ratio method is a common approach to determine the limit of quantitation. The concentration or the amount injected into the instrument corresponding to the signal – to – noise ratio of 10 : 1 is generally accepted.

4.6 Linearity

The linearity of an analytical method is its ability to elicit test results that are directly proportional to the concentration of analyte in sample within a given range.

Linearity relationship should be determined over the claimed range of the method. The samples with varying concentration of analyte for linearity determination are prepared by diluting accurately a stock solution, or by measuring accurately an amount of analyte separately. Five portions of samples should be prepared at least. The treatment is normally a calculation of a regression line by the method of least squares of test results versus analyte concentrations (when necessary). In some cases, the test data may have to be subjected to mathematical transformation prior to the linearity regression analysis.

Requirement for data: regression equation, correlation coefficient and the linear graph should be given.

4.7 Range

The range of an analytical method is the concentration or quantity internal between the upper and lower levels of analyte (including these levels) that have been demonstrated to be determined according to practical application and the results and demands of linearity, accuracy and precision. For toxic and special action compound, range should be more than the limit specified.

4.8 Ruggedness

Ruggedness of an analytical method is the degree of tolerance that the determination result is not affected when there is small change in the operational condition. The ruggedness of the method should be taken into account at the beginning to develop an analytical method. If the requirement for test condition is hard, it should be recorded clearly in the method. The typical variable factors are stability of the test solution, times and duration of sample extraction, and so on. The variable factors of liquid chromatography are composition and pH value of the mobile phase, same type of chromatography column but from different manufacturers or different batches, column temperature, flow rate, etc. The variable factors of GC are column and stationary phase with different brand or different batches, different type of support. Column temperature, sample inlet and detector temperature, etc.

It should be illustrated whether the testing conditions with slight change meet therequiments for system test to validate the method.

第四章 实验记录与报告

实验前应该认真预习，明确实验目的、原理和操作方法，并在实验记录本上写出扼要的预习记录（可用流程图等表示）和记录数据所需表格等。应及时记录实验过程中的各种测量数据及现象，不允许将数据记在小纸片上或随便记在其他地方。实验记录不能用铅笔，须用钢笔或圆珠笔。若发现数据读错、算错，而需要改动时，可将该数据用一横线划去，并在其下方或旁边写上正确的数据。中药分析实验报告一般包括以下内容：实验名称、日期、目的、原理和操作步骤。

一、实验记录和数据处理

（一）实验记录

记录内容一般包括供试药品名称、来源、批号、数量、规格、外观性状、包装情况、检验数据和结果等。记录数据时，要实事求是，决不能拼凑数据，要保留几位有效数字应和所用仪器的准确程度相适应。具体记录如下。

1. 鉴别实验

（1）显微鉴别　在实验中要画出特征显微结构并要有标注，描述特征显微结构要清晰明确如淀粉粒要写明是单粒还是复粒或者两者都有，大小、脐点、层纹崩裂或糊化等，草酸钙结晶要写明其晶形（方晶、柱晶、针晶、簇晶、沙晶等）、大小、结晶存在部位等，纤维和石细胞要描述其名称、性状、长度、细胞壁增厚情况等。

（2）理化鉴别　写明反应原理，描述清晰实验现象如燃烧反应要写明是否有黑烟还是白烟或无烟、爆鸣声等，荧光鉴别写明药材什么部位什么荧光颜色，沉淀反应写明沉淀的颜色，试管反应写明反应前后颜色变化等。

（3）薄层色鉴别　写明薄层色谱条件包括使用的薄层板、展开剂、显色剂、检视条件等，结果要绘制薄层色谱图标明样品和对照品位置。

2. 检查实验　写明检查项和原理，对于砷盐限量检查要写明用哪种砷盐检查方法及颜色变化，水分检查写明水分检查方法和所得数据等。

3. 含量测定　含量测定如果使用滴定法应记录滴定反应前后滴定管读数和颜色变化，使用 HPLC 法测定记录色谱条件，出峰时间，绘制色谱图，峰形情况等。

（二）数据处理

一般经过以下几方面。

1. 列表法　用表格将实验数据（包括原始数据与运算数值）记录出来就是列表法。实验数据列表本身就能直接反映有关量之间的关系。数据列表时的要求如下：①表格力求简单明了，分类清楚。②表中各量应写明单位，单位写在标题栏内，一般不要写在每个数字的后面。③表格中的数据要正确地表示出被测量的有效数字。

2. 作图法　标纸上描绘出所测一系列数据间关系的图线或通过计算机处理得到的图线就是作图法。该方法简便直观，易于揭示出物理量之间的变化规律，粗略显示出对应的函数关系。

二、实验报告

实验报告是做完每个实验后的总结。通过汇报本人的实验过程与结果，分析总结实验的经验和问题，加深对有关理论和技术的理解与掌握，同时也是学习撰写研究论文的基础。

1. 实验结果　应根据实验的要求将一定实验条件下获得的实验结果和数据进行整理、归纳、分析和对比，并尽量总结成各种图表，定性鉴别和检查实验要写明本次实验的结果如何，如定性鉴别要说明是否可检出被测成分、检查项目是否符合规定。

2. 问题与讨论　应对实验中实验方法（或操作技术）、观察的现象及实验结果进行分析和讨论，应对实验的正常结果和异常现象以及思考题进行探讨，对于实验设计的认识、体会和建议，如果实验失败，要寻找原因，总结经验教训，以提高自己的基本操作技能并对实验课提出的改进意见等。

Chapter 4　Experimental Record and Report

Before the experiment, students should be preview to get a basic knowledge of the purpose, basic principle and the method of the experiment, and write a brief preview report on the laboratory notebook, which can be indicated by the flow chart and the chart which needed to record the data. Various measurement data and phenomenon in the process of experiment, should be promptly recorded, do not allow the data recorded in a small piece of paper or casually down in other places, for the special requirements, according to the related provisions. The record of the experiment cannot use a pencil, use a pen or a ball pen, if you find the data read or calculated wrong, when modify is needed, a horizontal line can be drawn with the data, and write the correct below or beside. The report of Traditional Chinese Patent medicine (TCPM) analysis experiment including Experiment name, Experiment date, Experimental purpose (through this experiment to achieve the purpose of training), Basic principle (explain the principle by words, flow chart, reaction formula), operational procedure (described the operation steps should be concise and to the point).

1. Experimental record and data processing

(1) Experimental record　Record content should include the tested drug name, origin, batch number, quantity, specifications, appearance, packaging, the observed phenomenon, the results, etc. When record data, you should seek truth from facts, never piecing together the data, the effective number of bits (ENOB) should be in accordance with the accuracy of instrument. The records are as follows.

1) Identification test

①Microscopic identification: To draw the characteristics of microstructure and have a label. When describe the characteristics of microstructure, you should make clear that starch grains is single grain or composite grain or both, and specify the size, umbilical point, laminated crack or gelatinization. The calcium oxalate crystal should specify its crystalline form (solitary crystal, column needle crystal, clustered crystal, sand crystal etc.), its size and its location. The fiber and sclereid should describe its name, character, length, cell and the thickness of cell wall.

②The physicochemical identification: specify the reaction principle, clearly describe the experimental phenomena, such as the combustion reaction to specify whether it has black smoke and white smoke or smokeless, detonation. Fluorescent identification should specify the color of the fluorescence and at which part of the crude drugs. Precipitation reaction should specify the color of precipitation. Tube reaction should indicate the color changes before and after the reaction.

③TLC identification　Specify the thin layer chromatography conditions including thin layer plate, developing solvent, color developing agent, examination condition and etc. The results should draw a chromatography to indicate the position of samples and standard.

2) Examination   Specify the check items and principle, for arsenic salt limited inspection should specify what kind of arsenic salt inspection method was used and the color change, moisture inspection should indicate moisture inspection method and the result.

3) Content determination   Burette readings and color changes should be recorded before and after the titration reaction if titration was used. The chromatographic condition, retention, should be record if HPLC was used, and draw the chromatogram, spike, etc.

(2) Data processing   Data processing has the two parts.

1) The list method   With the form record experimental data (including raw data and Numerical Computing) is the list method; the list can reflect the relationship between the data. The following of requirement: ①the form should be simple and clear. ②The form should specify units, units written on the title bar, don't write on behind of every digital. ③The data should be significant digits in form.

2) The drawing method   Drawing on coordinate paper depicts the measured a series of relationships among data graphs or through computer processing line is the drawing method. The method is simple and intuitive, easy to reveal the change law between physical quantities, roughly show the functional relation.

2. Experimental report

The experimental report is the summary of the experiment. Through reporting the experimental process and the result, analyzing and summarizing the experience and problems of experiment, it can deepen our understanding and mastering of the related theory and techniques, and it is also the process of learning to write a research paper.

(1) The experimental results   According to different experimental requirements, we should conclude, analysis and compare the date and the result obtained in the certain experimental conditions, and try to tabulate. The qualitative identification and examination experiment should indicate what the result, such as qualitative identification should indicate it whether can detect the checked components and the checked item whether meet the specification.

(2) The question and discussion   Analysis and discuss the experimental method, the phenomena and the experimental results (no matter the reasonable results or the abnormal phenomena). To the understanding experimental design, you should have a deep understanding. You also should find the reasons; sum up the lessons learned if the experiment failed, so you can improve the basic operating skills. And you may also provide the valuable advice for curriculum improvement.

第二部分 各类中药分析实验

Part 2 Various Kinds of Experiment for Analysis of Traditional Chinese Medicine

第五章 单项实验

Chapter 5 Individual Experiment

实验一 五苓散与万氏牛黄清心丸的显微鉴别

【目的要求】

1. 熟悉中药制剂的显微鉴别方法。

2. 掌握丸剂显微鉴别的目的、原理及操作方法。

【原理】

利用由药材粉末组成的中药制剂保留原药材的组织、细胞或内含物等显微特征以鉴别中药制剂的处方。

【仪器、试剂与药品】

1. **仪器** 显微镜、偏光显微镜、离心机。

2. **材料** 载玻片、盖玻片、小镊子、小刀、酒精灯、乳钵、擦镜纸。

3. **试剂** 水合氯醛试液、甘油醋酸试液、稀甘油。

4. **药品** 五苓散（市售品）、万氏牛黄清心丸（市售品）。

【实验内容】

1. 五苓散的鉴别 取本品少许，用甘油醋酸试液装片，观察淀粉粒和不规则分枝状团块；另取少许用水合氯醛试液透化后滴加适量稀甘油，置显微镜下观察。

2. 万氏牛黄清心丸的鉴别 取本品 2 丸，切碎，加热水搅拌、洗涤后，置离心管中离心分离沉淀（或自然沉降），滤过，取少许滤渣，用甘油醋酸试液装片，观察糊化淀粉粒；另取少许滤渣用水合氯醛试液透化后滴加适量稀甘油，置显微镜下观察。

【实验记录】

1. 记录五苓散的鉴别实验结果，绘制显微鉴别图。

2. 记录万氏牛黄清心丸的鉴别实验结果，绘制显微鉴别图。

【思考题】

1. 试述观察到的显微特征，各代表何种中药材？

2. 通过以上实验，试总结出中药制剂显微鉴别的方法及注意事项。

【相关资料】

1. **五苓散的处方** 茯苓 180g，泽泻 300g，猪苓 180g，肉桂 120g，白术（炒）180g。制法：以上五味，粉碎成细粉，过筛，混匀，即得。功能与主治：温阳化气，利湿行水。用于阳不化气、水湿内停所致的水肿，症见小便不利、水肿腹胀、呕逆泄泻、渴不思饮。

2. **万氏牛黄清心丸的处方** 牛黄 10g，朱砂 60g，黄连 200g，黄芩 120g，栀子 120g，郁金 80g。制法：以上六味，除牛黄外，朱砂水飞成极细粉；其余黄连等四味粉碎成细粉；将牛黄研细，与上述粉末配研，过筛，混匀，每 100g 粉末加炼蜜 100～120g 制成大蜜丸，即得。功能与主治：清热解毒，镇惊安神。用于热入心包、热盛动风证，症见高热烦躁、神昏谵语及小儿高热惊厥。

3. **五苓散显微鉴别** 茯苓的粉末特征为不规则分枝状团块无色，遇水合氯醛液溶化；菌丝无色，直径 4～6μm。猪苓的粉末特征为菌丝黏结成团，大多无色；草酸钙方晶正八面体形，直径 32～60μm。泽泻的粉末特征为薄壁细胞类圆形，有椭圆形纹孔，集成纹孔群。炒白术的粉末特征为草酸钙针晶细小，长 10～32μm，不规则地充塞于薄壁细胞中。肉桂的粉末特征为纤维单个散在，长梭形，直径 24～50μm，壁厚，木化；石细胞类方形或类圆形，壁一面菲薄（图 5 – 1）。

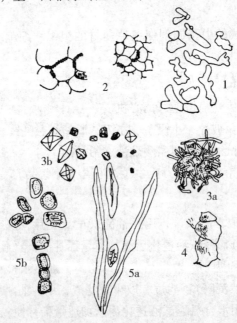

图 5 – 1 五苓散的显微鉴别图

1. 茯苓（分枝状团块） 2. 泽泻（薄壁细胞） 3. 猪苓（a. 菌丝黏结成团；b. 草酸钙晶体） 4. 炒白术（草酸钙针晶） 5. 肉桂（a. 纤维；b. 石细胞）

4. 万氏牛黄清心丸显微鉴别 郁金的粉末特征为糊化淀粉粒团块，几乎无色。栀子的粉末特征为种皮石细胞黄色或淡棕色，多破碎，完整者长多角形、长方形或形状不规则，壁厚，呈瘤状伸入胞腔，孔沟末端常膨大呈圆囊状，胞腔及孔沟含棕色物。黄芩的粉末特征为韧皮纤维淡黄色，梭形，壁厚，孔沟细。黄连的粉末特征为石细胞鲜黄色，类方形、类圆形、类长方形或多角形，壁稍厚，纹孔明显。朱砂的粉末特征为不规则细小颗粒暗棕红色，有光泽，边缘暗黑色（图5-2）。

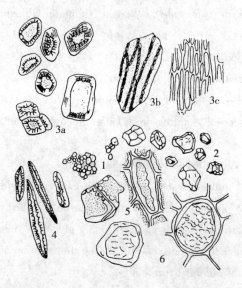

图5-2 万氏牛黄清心丸的显微鉴别图

1. 人工牛黄（黄色色素及淀粉粒） 2. 朱砂 3. 黄连（a. 石细胞；b. 木纤维；c. 磷叶表皮细胞表面观） 4. 黄芩（韧皮纤维） 5. 栀子（种皮石细胞） 6. 郁金（含糊化淀粉粒细胞）

5. 试剂的配制

（1）水合氯醛试液 取水合氯醛50g，加水15ml与甘油10ml使溶解，即得。

（2）甘油醋酸试液 取甘油、50%醋酸与水各等份，混合，即得。

Experiment 1 Microscopical Identification of Wuling Powder and Wanshi Niuhuang Qingxin Pills

Purpose

1. To be familiar with the method of the microscopical identification of traditional Chinese patent medicine.

2. To master the purpose, principle and operation of the microscopical identification for pills.

Principle

As each drug in these two patents retains the powder characters of the crude drug, we can identify them by the means of microscopical identification through observing microscopical characters of tissues, cells or cell contents of crude drugs.

Apparatus, materials, reagents and drugs

1. Apparatus: microscope, polarization microscope, centrifuge.

2. Materials: slide, cover glass, tweezer, shaver, alcohol burner, mortar, paper for erasing lens.

3. Reagents: chloralhydrate TS, glycerin – acetic acid TS, glycerin dilute TS.

4. Drugs: Wuling Powder (for sale), Wanshi Niuhuang Qingxin Pills (for sale).

Experiment contents

1. Identification of Wuling Powder

To a small quantity of the patent, starch granules and irregular branched masses can be observed by using glycerin – acetic acid TS asmountant; other microscopical characters can be observed under the microscope by adding dropwise an adequate quantity of dilute glycerin after the disposal of chloral hydrate TS.

2. Identification of Wanshi Niuhuang Pills

To 2 pills, in pieces, add hot water, stir and wash, then transfer into a centrifugal tube, centrifuge and separate the precipitate (or naturally subside), filter, to a small quantity of the filter residue, observe gelatinized starch granules using glycerin – acetic acid TS asmountant, others can be observed under the microscope by adding dropwise an adequate quantity of dilute glycerin after the disposal of chloral hydrate TS.

Experiment records

1. Record the microscopical identification test result of Wuling powder and draw the micrograph.

2. Record the microscopical identification test result of Wanshi Niuhuang Pills and draw the micrograph.

Questions

1. Try to describe the microscopical characters observed. Which drug does each of them stand for?

2. Through the above experiment, please summarize the methods of microscopical identification of Traditional Chinese Medicine Preparation and their precautions?

Related materials

1. Ingredients of Wuling powder   Poria 180 g, Alismatis Rhizoma 300 g, Polyporus 180 g, Cinnamomi Cotex 120 g, Atractylodis Macrocephalae phalae Rhizoma (stir – baked) 180 g. Procedure: Pulverize the above five ingredients to fine powder, sift and mix. Action: To warm yang and promote qi transformation, and drain dampness and move water. Indications: Edema caused by yang failing to transform qi and internal water – dampness retention, manifested as inhibited urination, edema, abdominal distension, vomiting and hiccup, diarrhea and thirst with no desire for drinks.

2. Ingredients of Wanshi Niuhuang Qingxin Pills   Bovis Calculus 10 g, Cinnabaris 60 g,

Coptidis Rhizoma 200 g, Scutellariae Radix 120 g, Gardeniae Fructus 120 g, Curcumae Radix 80 g. Procedure: Levigate Cinnabaris to very fine powder, and pulverize Coptidis Rhizoma, Gardeniae Fructus and Curcumae Radix to fine powder. Triturate Bovis with the above five ingredients, sift and mix well. To each 100 g of the powder add 100 – 120 g of refined honey to make big honeyed pills. Action: To clear heat and remove toxin, settle fright and stabilize mind. Indications: Pattern of heat entering the pericardium and exuberant heat stirring – up wind, manifested as vexation and restlessness in high fever; loss of consciousness and delirious speech; fright syncope in children caused by high fever.

3. For Wuling Powder, microscopical of Poria is irregular branched masses colourless, dissolved in chloral hydrate TS; hyphae colourless or brownish, 4 – 6 μm in diameter. Microscopical of Polyporus is hyphae sticking into masses, mostly colourless; prisms of calcium oxalate octahedral, 32 – 60 μm in diameter. Microscopical of Alismatis Rhizoma is parenchymatous cells subrounded, with elliptical pits gathered into pit groups. Microscopical of Atractylodis Macrocephalae phalae Rhizoma is needle crystals of calcium oxalate fine, 10 – 32 μm long, irregularly filling in parenchymatous cells. Microscopical of Cinnamomi Cortex is fibre singly scattered, long fusiform, 24 – 50 μm in diameter, walls thickened, lignified; stone cells subsquare or subrounded, with thinner walls on one side（Figure 5 – 1）.

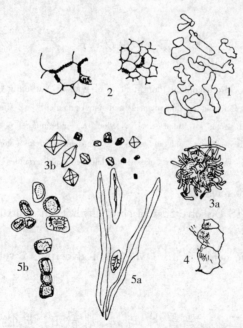

Figure 5 – 1　Microscopical Identification of Wuling Powder

1. Poria（irregular branched masses）　2. Alismatis Rhizoma（parenchymatous cells）

3. Polyporus（a. hyphae sticking into masses；b. prisms of calcium oxalate）

4. Atractylodis Macrocephalae phalae Rhizoma（needle crystals of calcium oxalate）

5. Cinnamomi Cortex（a. fibre；b. stone cells）

4. For Wanshi Niuhuang Qingxin Pills, microscopical of Curcumae Radix is masses of ge-

latinised starch granules almost colourless. Microscopical of Gardeniae Fructus is stone cells of testa yellow or brownish, mostly broken, when whole, long polygonal, rectangular or irregular, walls thickened, with large rounded pits, the lumina containing brownish – red contents. Microscopical of Scutellariae Radix is phloem fibres pale yellow, fusiform with thickened walls and fine pit – canals. Microscopical of Coptidis Rhizomais stone cells bright yellow, with slightly thickened walls and distinct pits. Microscopical of Cinnabaris is irregular minute granules dark brown, lustrous, and with dark black edges (Figure 5 – 2).

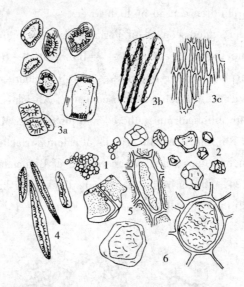

Figure 5 – 2　Microscopical Identification of Wanshi Niuhuang Qingxin Pills

1. Bovis Calculus (yellow pigments and starch granules)　　2. Cinnabaris

3. Coptidis Rhizoma (a. stone cells; b. xylon, c. epidermic cell of scale leaf)

4. Scutellariae Radix (phloem fibres)　　5. Gardeniae Fructus (stone cells)

6. Curcumae Radix (masses of gelatinised starch granules)

5. The preparation of reagents

(1) Chloralhydrate TS　Dissolve 50 g of choral hydrate in a mixture of 15 ml of water and 10 ml of glycerin.

(2) Glycerin – acetic acid TS　Mix 1 volume of glycerin, 1 volume of 50% acetic acid and 1 volume of water.

实验二　安胃片与冰硼散的理化鉴别

【目的要求】

1. 熟悉中药制剂的一般理化鉴别方法。

2. 掌握一般理化鉴别的目的、原理及操作方法。

【原理】

采用一般理化鉴别方法（如化学反应法、升华法等）鉴别处方。安胃片中延胡索所含生物碱在紫外光下能产生亮黄绿色荧光；煅白矾中的硫酸铝钾$KAl(SO_4)_2$显铝盐和硫酸盐的鉴别反应；海螵蛸中的碳酸钙（$CaCO_3$）显钙盐和碳酸盐的鉴别反应。

冰硼散中冰片即龙脑，可与香草醛硫酸溶液反应，显紫色；玄明粉中的无水硫酸钠（Na_2SO_4）显硫酸盐的鉴别反应；朱砂中的硫化汞（HgS），显汞盐反应；硼砂中的四硼酸钠（$Na_2B_4O_7 \cdot 10H_2O$）显硼酸盐的鉴别反应。

【仪器、试剂与药品】

1. **仪器** 恒温水浴锅、三用紫外线分析仪、分析天平。

2. **材料** 冷凝管（24#）、圆底烧瓶（24#，250ml）、乳钵、滤纸、姜黄试纸、小漏斗、具塞试管（10ml）、量筒（10ml）、试管、烧杯、毛细管、干燥小瓶、蒸发皿、钢铲、铜片。

3. **试剂与试药** 乙醇、乙醚、蒸馏水、5%氢氧化钠、5%氢氧化钙、氨水、10%草酸铵、稀盐酸、10%醋酸、5%硝酸、10%亚硝酸钴钠试液、饱和氯化钡试液、1%香草醛硫酸溶液。

4. **药品** 安胃片（市售品）；冰硼散（市售品）。

【实验内容】

1. 安胃片的鉴别

（1）取本品2片，研细，置试管中，加稀盐酸10ml，即泡沸，放出二氧化碳气体，气体遇氢氧化钙试液，即生成白色沉淀。将试管中的酸性液体滤过，取滤液3ml，加氨试液使成微碱性，即生成白色胶状沉淀，滤过，沉淀在盐酸、醋酸或过量的氢氧化钠试液中溶解；滤液中加草酸铵试液2滴，即生成白色沉淀，在盐酸中溶解，但在醋酸中不溶。

（2）取本品2片，研细，置小烧杯中，加水10ml，充分搅拌，滤过。取滤液2ml，加氯化钡试液2滴，即生成白色沉淀，在盐酸或硝酸中均不溶解；另取滤液2ml，加亚硝酸钴钠试液2滴，即生成黄色沉淀。

2. 冰硼散的鉴别

（1）取本品1g，加水6ml，振摇，加盐酸使成酸性后，滤过，分取滤液3ml，点于姜黄试纸上使润湿，即显橙红色，放置干燥，颜色变深，置氨蒸气中熏，变为绿黑色。

（2）取（1）项的剩余滤液，加氯化钡试液1～2滴，即生成白色沉淀，分离后，沉淀在盐酸中不溶解。

（3）取本品1g，置试管中，加水10ml，用力振摇，在试管底部很快出现朱红色的沉淀，分取少量沉淀用盐酸湿润，在光洁的铜片上摩擦，铜片表面即显银白色光泽，加热烘烤后银白色即消失。

（4）取本品0.5g，加乙醚10ml，振摇，滤过，滤液置蒸发皿中，放置，待乙醚挥发后，加新配制的1%香草醛硫酸溶液1～2滴，显紫色。

【实验记录】

1. 记录实验过程中出现的现象。

2. 记录实验过程中出现的问题并说明可能的原因。

【思考题】

1. 试述各鉴别步骤的化学定性原理是什么？分别用于鉴定处方中的哪味药？

2. 如何提高理化鉴别方法的专属性？

【相关资料】

1. **安胃片**　处方：醋制延胡索63g，煅白矾250g，去壳海螵蛸187g。制法：以上三味，粉碎成细粉，过筛，混匀，加蜂蜜125g与适量的水，制成颗粒，干燥，压制成1000片，即得。功能与主治：行气活血，制酸止痛。用于气滞血瘀所致的胃脘刺痛、吞酸嗳气、脘闷不舒；胃及十二指肠溃疡、慢性胃炎见上述证候者。

2. **冰硼散**　处方：冰片50g，煅硼砂500g，朱砂60g，玄明粉500g。制法：以上四味，朱砂水飞成极细粉，硼砂粉碎成细粉，将冰片研细，与上述粉末及玄明粉配研，过筛，混匀，即得。功能与主治：清热解毒，消肿止痛。用于热毒蕴结所致的咽喉疼痛、牙龈肿痛、口舌生疮。

3. **中药制剂的理化鉴别**　是指利用物理、化学的方法对其所含的化学成分进行定性鉴别，从而判断中药制剂的真伪。目前一般理化鉴别方法有：化学反应法、升华法和光谱法等。

化学反应法是选择适宜的化学反应和试剂，从反应后颜色的变化、沉淀的生成等现象鉴别真伪。但要慎重使用专属性不好的化学反应，如泡沫生成反应、三氯化铁显色反应等，因为中药材中蛋白质、含酚性羟基等类似成分的存在较为普遍。在分析前应对样品进行分离、精制，除去干扰鉴别反应的物质，借此改善鉴别方法的专属性。采用阴性对照和阳性对照的方式，对拟定的鉴别方法进行反复验证，防止出现假阳性。

升华法是利用中药中所含的某些化学成分，在一定温度下能升华的性质，获得升华物，在显微镜下观察其结晶形状、颜色及化学反应，适用于含有升华性成分药材（如大黄、牡丹皮、冰片、薄荷、安息香、斑蝥等）的成药。

可见－紫外分光光度法是利用中药材中有些化学成分在可见紫外光区有选择性吸收，显示特征吸收光谱，以鉴别中药制剂中的某些成分。需注意中药制剂组成复杂，成分众多，根据吸收度的加和性，当样品不经纯化时，所得光谱为混合光谱，专属性差。为了提高本法的专属性，可选择适当的方法将样品纯化后测定吸收光谱。

4. **稀盐酸的配制**　取盐酸234ml，加水稀释至1000ml，即得。

Experiment 2　Physical – Chemical Identification of

Anwei Tablets and Bingpeng Powder

Purpose

1. To be acquainted with method of physical and chemical identification.

2. To master the purpose, principle and method of physical and chemical identification.

Principle

Identify the ingredients of Traditional Chinese Medicine Preparation by physical and chemical identification method (e. g. chemical reaction method and sublimation). Since Rhizoma Corydalis in Anwei Tablets contains alkaloids which show bright yellowish – green fluorescence under ultraviolet light, it can be identified accordingly. The main constituent of Alumen (calcined), $KAl (SO_4)_2$, shows positive reaction of aluminum salt and sulfate. Endoconcha Sepiae mainly contains $CaCO_3$, which can be identified by the reaction of calcium salt and carbonate.

Borneolum Syntheticum (borneol) in Bingpeng Powder shows purple colour after react with vanillin in sulfuric acid. The main composition of Borax, Na_2SO_4, shows positive reaction of sulfate. Cinnabaris mainly contains HgS, which can be identified by the reaction of mercuric salt. Natrii Sulfas Exsiccatus contains $Na_2B_4O_7 \cdot 10H_2O$, which shows positive reaction of borate.

Apparatus, materials, reagents and drugs

1. Apparatus: water bath, ultraviolet analyzer, analytical balance.

2. Materials: condenser pipe ($24^{\#}$), round bottom flask ($24^{\#}$, 250 ml), mortar, filter paper, tumeric paper, small funnel, test tube (10 ml), small beaker, capillaries, drying small flask, evaporating dish, steel fork, smooth copper plate.

3. Reagents: ethanol, ether, re – distilled water, 5% sodium hydroxide TS, 5% calcium hydroxide TS, ammonia TS, 10% ammonium oxalate TS, dilute hydrochloric acid, 10% acetic acid TS, 5% nitric acid, 10% sodium cobalt nitrite TS, saturated barium chloride TS, 1% vanillin in sulfuric acid.

4. Drugs: Anwei Tablets (for sale); Bingpeng Powder (for sale).

Experiment contents

1. Identification of Anwei Tablets

(1) Place 2 tablets, in fine powder, in a test tube, add 10 ml of dilute hydrochloric acid, it effervesces and evolves carbon dioxide, which produces a white precipitate on introducing into calcium hydroxide TS. Filter the acidic solution in the test tube. Transfer 3 ml of the filtrate, alkalize slightly with ammonia TS, a white colloid precipitate is produced, which is soluble in hydrochloric acid TS, acetic acid TS and in an excess of sodium hydroxide TS. To

the filtrate add 2 drops of ammonium oxalate TS, a white precipitate is produced, which is soluble in hydrochloric acid, but insoluble in acetic acid.

(2) Place 2 tablets, in fine powder, in a small beaker, add 10 ml of water, stir thoroughly and filter. To 2 ml of the filtrate add 2 drops of barium chloride TS, a white precipitate is produced, which is insoluble in hydrochloric acid or nitric acid. To another 2 ml of the filtrate add 2 drop of sodium cobalt nitrite TS; a yellow precipitate is produced.

2. Identification of Bingpeng Powder

(1) To 1 g add 6 ml of water, shake, acidify with hydrochloric acid and filter. Moisten a strip of tumeric paper with 3 ml of the filtrate, an orange – red colour is produced, the colour darkens on dryness and turns greenish – black on exposure to ammonia vapour.

(2) To the remained filtrate obtained under Identification test (1), add 1 – 2 drops of barium chloride TS, a white precipitate is produced, which, after separating, is insoluble in hydrochloric acid.

(3) Place 1 g in a test tube, add 10 ml of water and shake vigorously, a vermilion precipitate is rapidly produced at the bottom of the test tube. Separate a small quantity of the precipitate, moisten with hydrochloric acid, rub on a smooth copper plate, a silver lustre is produced, and disappears on heating.

(4) To 0. 5 g add 10 ml of ether, shake and filter. Transfer the filtrate to an evaporating dish, evaporate the ether on standing and to the residue add 1 – 2 drops of freshly prepared 1% solution of vanillin in sulfuric acid, a purple colour is produced.

Experiment records

1. Record the phenomena of the experiment.

2. Make a record of the problems appeared during the experiment and illuminate the causes of the problems.

Questions

1. Please describe the chemical qualitative principle of each identification experiment, which drug does each identification identify in these patents?

2. How to improve the specialist of physical and chemical identification?

Related materials

1. Ingredients of Anwei Tablets   Corydalis Rhizoma (processed with vinegar) 63 g, Alumen (calcined) 250 g, Sepiae Endoconcha 187 g. Procedure: Pulverize the above three ingredients to fine powder, sift and mix well. Make granules with 125 g of honey and a quantity of water, dry, compress into 1000 tablets. Action: To move qi and activate blood, inhibit acidity and relieve pain. Indications: Stomach stabbing pain, acid regurgitation and belching, oppression and epigastric discomfort caused by qi stagnation and blood stasis; Gastroduodenal ulcer and chronic gastritis with pattern mentioned above.

2. Ingredients of Bingpeng Powder   Borneolum Syntheticum 50 g, Borax (calcined) 500 g, Cinnabaris 60 g, Natrii Sulfas Exsiccatus 500 g. Procedure: Levigate Cinnabaris to very fine

powder, pulverize Borax to fine powder and triturate Borneolum Syntheticum with the above powders and Natrii Sulfas Exsiccatus, sift and mix well. Action: To clear heat, remove toxicity, disperse swelling, relieve pain. Indications: Sore throat, swelling painful gum, mouth and tongue sore caused by accumulated heat toxin.

3. The physical and chemical identification of Traditional Chinese Medicine Preparationis used physical and chemical methods to identify the chemical composition in patent so that the patent can be identified. Now the usual methods of physical and chemical identification are chemical reaction method, sublimation, spectrometry and so on.

Chemical reaction method is the method of choosing suitable chemical reaction and reagent to produce colour changing, precipitate and other phenomena to identify the patents. Avoiding to use the reaction with poor specialist, e. g. foam aroused reaction, ferric chloride colour reaction, for many traditional Chinese medicines contain protein and compounds possessing phenolic hydroxyl group. The sample must be separated and purified to eliminate disturbing substance so that the identification method has a better specialist. The identification method must be validated by negative and positive comparison to avoid fake positive phenomena.

Sublimation is the method according to the character of compounds which can sublimate at certain temperature in Chinese drug, and the crystal shape, colour and colour reaction of sublimation can be observed under microscope. The method is suitable to the patents which have drugs containing sublimated substances (e. g. Rhei Radix et Rhizoma, Moutan Cortex, Borneolum, Menthae Herba, Benzoinum, Mylabris).

Ultraviolet – visible spectrophotometry is a method according to the character of compound in traditional Chinese medicine which has selective absorption in Ultraviolet – visible light range, shows characteristic absorption spectrum so that Traditional Chinese Medicine Preparationcontaining the traditional Chinese medicine can be identified. When using spectrum method to identify Traditional Chinese patent medicine, we often get mixed spectrum since the samples have not been purified, so it need to be purified by suitable method before identifying absorption spectrum.

4. The preparation of hydrochloric acid dilute TS　Dilute 234 ml of hydrochloric acid with water to 1000 ml.

实验三　桂枝茯苓丸与葛根芩连片的薄层色谱鉴别

【目的要求】
1. 熟悉中药制剂的薄层色谱鉴别方法。
2. 掌握薄层色谱鉴别的目的、原理及操作方法。
【原理】
利用薄层色谱法，以对照品和对照药材作对照鉴别中药制剂的处方。

【仪器、试剂与药品】

1. **仪器** 三用紫外线分析仪、分析天平（0.1mg）、超声波清洗器。

2. **材料** 双槽层析缸、玻璃板5cm×12cm、量筒（10ml、25ml）、移液管（5ml、1ml）。

3. **试剂** 甲醇、乙醇、无水乙醇、异丙醇、正丁醇、三氯甲烷、甲苯、丁酮、氨水、乙醚、乙酸乙酯、石油醚（60~90℃）、环己烷、甲酸、盐酸、二硝基苯肼乙醇试液、盐酸酸性5%三氯化铁乙醇溶液、5%香草醛硫酸溶液、2%三氯化铁乙醇、含0.3%的羧甲基纤维素钠为黏合剂的硅胶G的薄层板。

4. **药品** 桂皮醛对照品乙醇溶液（1μg/ml）、丹皮酚对照品乙醇溶液（1mg/ml）、芍药苷对照品乙醇溶液（1mg/ml）、盐酸小檗碱对照品甲醇溶液（0.5mg/ml）、葛根素对照品无水乙醇溶液（1mg/ml）、黄芩苷对照品甲醇溶液（1mg/ml）；黄连对照药材；桂枝茯苓丸（市售品）、葛根芩连片（市售品）。

【实验内容】

1. 桂枝茯苓丸的鉴别

（1）桂枝的鉴别

1）供试品溶液制备 取本品6g，切碎，加乙醚50ml，低温加热回流1小时，滤过，药渣备用，滤液低温挥去乙醚，残渣加乙醇1ml使溶解，作为供试品溶液。

2）薄层色谱条件及方法 吸取供试品溶液10μl、桂皮醛对照品乙醇溶液3μl，分别点于同一硅胶G薄层板上，以石油醚（60~90℃）-乙酸乙酯（17:3）为展开剂，展开，取出，晾干，喷以二硝基苯肼乙醇试液。供试品色谱中，在与对照品色谱相应的位置上，显相同颜色的斑点。

（2）牡丹皮的鉴别

1）供试品溶液的制备 取"桂枝的鉴别"项下的供试液。

2）薄层色谱条件及方法 吸取"桂枝的鉴别"项下的供试品溶液及丹皮酚对照品乙醇溶液各10μl，分别点于同一硅胶G薄层板上，以环己烷-乙酸乙酯（3:1）为展开剂，展开，取出，晾干，喷以盐酸酸性5%三氯化铁乙醇溶液，加热至斑点显色清晰。供试品色谱中，在与对照品色谱相应的位置上，显相同颜色的斑点。

（3）赤芍的鉴别

1）供试品溶液的制备 取"桂枝的鉴别"项下的备用药渣，加乙醇20ml，超声处理15分钟，滤过，滤液蒸干，残渣加水15ml使溶解，用以水饱和的正丁醇振摇提取2次，每次20ml，合并正丁醇液，用水洗涤2次，每次10ml，弃去水洗液，将正丁醇液置水浴上蒸干，残渣加乙醇1ml使溶解，作为供试品溶液。

2）薄层色谱条件及方法 吸取供试品溶液10μl、芍药苷对照品乙醇溶液5μl，分别点于同一硅胶G薄层板上，以三氯甲烷-乙酸乙酯-甲醇-甲酸（40:5:10:0.2）为展开剂，展开，取出，晾干，喷以5%香草醛硫酸溶液，加热至斑点显色清晰。供试品色谱中，在与对照品色谱相应的位置上，显相同的蓝紫色斑点。

2. 葛根芩连片的鉴别

（1）黄连的鉴别

1）供试品溶液制备　取本品 2 片，研细，加甲醇 10ml，超声处理 15 分钟，滤过，取滤液 1ml，用甲醇稀释至 5ml，作为供试品溶液。

2）对照药材溶液的制备　取黄连对照药材 0.1g，加甲醇 10ml，超声处理 15 分钟，滤过，滤液作为对照药材溶液。

3）薄层色谱条件及方法　吸取上述两种溶液及盐酸小檗碱对照品甲醇溶液各 1μl，分别点于同一硅胶 G 薄层板上，以甲苯 – 乙酸乙酯 – 甲醇 – 异丙醇 – 浓氨试液（12:6:3:3:1）为展开剂，置氨蒸气预饱和 15 分钟的展开缸内，展开，取出，晾干，置紫外光灯（365nm）下检视。供试品色谱中，在与对照药材色谱及对照品色谱相应的位置上，显相同颜色的荧光斑点。

（2）葛根的鉴别

1）供试品溶液制备　取本品 4 片，研细，加乙酸乙酯 25ml，超声处理 30 分钟，滤过，滤液蒸干，残渣加甲醇 0.5ml 使溶解，作为供试品溶液。

2）薄层色谱条件及方法　吸取供试品溶液 5μl、对照品溶液 2μl，分别点于同一硅胶 G 薄层板上，以三氯甲烷 – 甲醇 – 水（28:10:1）为展开剂，展开，取出，晾干，置氨蒸气中熏 15 分钟，置紫外光灯（365nm）下检视。供试品色谱中，在与对照品色谱相应的位置上，显相同颜色的荧光斑点。

（3）黄芩的鉴别

1）薄层板制备　含 4% 醋酸钠的羧甲基纤维素钠溶液为黏合剂的硅胶 G 的薄层板（实验前自制）。

2）供试品溶液制备　取本品 4 片，研细，加甲醇 30ml，加热回流 30 分钟，滤过，滤液蒸干，残渣加水 10ml 使溶解，加盐酸调节 pH 至 3.0 ~ 3.5，用乙酸乙酯振摇提取 2 次，每次 10ml，合并提取液，蒸干，残渣加甲醇 1ml 使溶解，作为供试品溶液。

3）薄层色谱条件及方法　吸取供试品溶液 10μl、对照品溶液 5μl，分别点于同一含 4% 醋酸钠的羧甲基纤维素钠溶液为黏合剂的硅胶 G 薄层板上，以乙酸乙酯 – 丁酮 – 甲酸 – 水（5:3:1:1）为展开剂，展开，取出，晾干，喷以 2% 三氯化铁乙醇溶液。供试品色谱中，在与对照品色谱相应的位置上，显相同颜色的荧光斑点。

【实验记录】

1. 记录桂枝茯苓丸的鉴别实验结果，绘制薄层色谱图并算出主要斑点的 R_f 值。

2. 记录葛根芩连片的鉴别实验结果，绘制薄层色谱图并算出主要斑点的 R_f 值。

【思考题】

1. 在薄层色谱鉴别中，常用显色剂有哪些？分别用于鉴别哪类成分？

2. 鉴别葛根芩连片中的黄连时，为什么使用氨蒸气预饱和展开缸？

3. 鉴别葛根芩连片中的黄芩时，为什么在硅胶 G 中，加入 4% 醋酸钠？

【相关资料】

1. 桂枝茯苓丸　处方：桂枝 100g，茯苓 100g，牡丹皮 100g，赤芍 100g，桃仁 100g。制法：以上五味，粉碎成细粉，过筛，混匀。每 100g 粉末加炼蜜 90 ~ 110g 制成大蜜丸，即得。功能与主治：活血，化瘀，消癥。用于妇人宿有癥块，或血瘀经闭，行经腹痛，产后恶露不尽。

2. 葛根芩连片 处方：葛根 1000g，黄芩 375g，黄连 375g，炙甘草 250g。制法：以上四味，取葛根 225g，粉碎成细粉，剩余的葛根与甘草加水煎煮两次，每次 2 小时，合并煎液，滤过，滤液适当浓缩；黄芩和黄连分别用 50% 乙醇作溶剂，浸渍 24 小时后进行渗漉，收集渗漉液，回收乙醇后与上述浓缩液合并，浓缩成稠膏状，加入葛根细粉，混匀，干燥，制成颗粒，干燥，压制成 1000 片，即得。功能与主治：解肌清热，止泻止痢。用于湿热蕴结所致的泄泻、痢疾，症见身热烦渴、下痢臭秽、腹痛不适。

3. 桂枝茯苓丸中主要成分 在桂枝茯苓丸中，桂皮醛（cinnamyl aldehyde）是桂枝挥发油中的主要成分，另含醋酸桂皮酯（cinnamyl acetate）、桂皮酸（cinnamic acid）等成分。

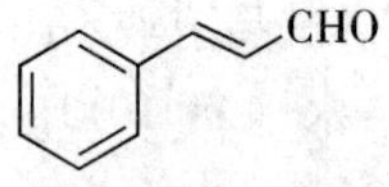

桂皮醛

牡丹皮的主要成分为丹皮酚（paeonol），此外，尚含牡丹酚原苷（paeonolide）、牡丹酚苷（paeonoside）等成分。

赤芍主含芍药苷（paeoniflorin），另含少量羟基芍药苷（oxypaeoniflorin）、苯甲酰芍药苷（benzoylpaeoniflorin）等成分。

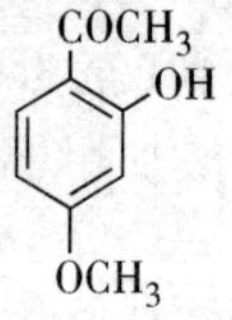

丹皮酚 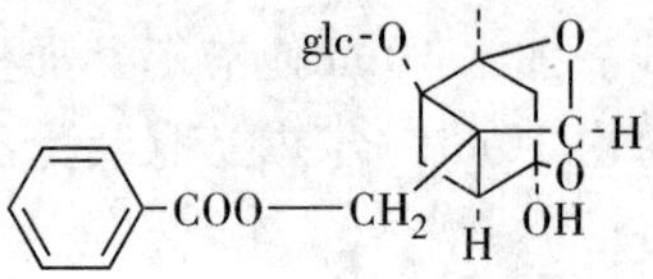   芍药苷

4. 葛根芩连片中主要成分 在葛根芩连片中，葛根含多种异黄酮类成分，含量约为 12%，其中，主要为葛根素（葛根黄素，puerarin）、黄豆苷（daidzin）等。

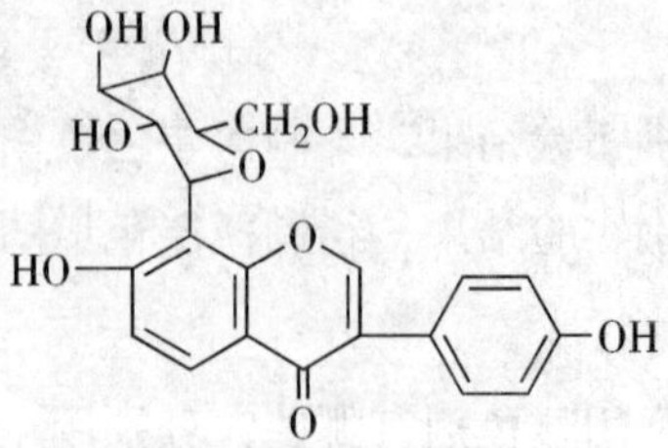

葛根素

黄芩苷（baicalin）为黄芩的主要有效成分，在黄芩中的含量为 4% ~ 5%。黄芩含多种黄酮类化合物，其他如汉黄芩苷（wogonoside）、千层纸素 A 葡萄糖醛酸苷（oroxylin glucuronide）等。

黄芩苷

5. 二硝基苯肼乙醇试液的配制　取 2，4 - 二硝基苯肼 1g，加乙醇 1000ml 使溶解，再缓缓加入盐酸 10ml，摇匀，即得。

Experiment 3　Identification of Guizhi Fuling Pills and Gegen Qinlian Tablets by TLC

Purpose

1. To be acquainted with the method of the identification of traditional Chinese patent medicines by TLC.

2. To master the purpose, theory and operation of identification by TLC.

Principle

Thin layer chromatography is used to identify traditional Chinese patent medicines in comparison with reference substances and reference drugs.

Apparatus, materials, reagents and drugs

1. Apparatus: three - purpose ultraviolet analyser, analytical balance (0.1 mg), ultrasonic surge.

2. Materials: double groove chromatographic chamber, glass plate 5 cm × 12 cm, graduated cylinder (10 ml, 25 ml), transfer pipette (5 ml, 1 ml).

3. Reagents: methanol, ethanol, dehydrated ethanol, isopropanol, *n* - butanol, chloroform, toluene, butanone, ammonia solution, ethyl acetate, petroleum ether (60 - 90℃), cyclohexane, formic acid, hydrochloric acid, 2% ferric chloride in ethanol, dinitrophenylhydrazine TS in ethanol, 5% ferric chloride in ethanol acidated with hydrochloric acid, 5% vanillin in sulfuric acid, Silica gel G prepared with 0.3% sodium carboxymethyl - cellulose solution (coating before experiment).

4. Drugs: cinnamaldehyde CRS in ethanol (1μg/ml), paeonol CRS in ethanol (1 mg/ml), paeoniflorin CRS in ethanol (1 mg/ml), berberine hydrochloride CRS in methanol (0.5 mg/ml), puerarin CRS in dehydrated ethanol (1 mg/ml), baicalin CRS; Rhizoma Coptidis reference drug; Guizhi Fuling Pills (for sale) and Gegen Qinlian Tablets (for sale).

Experiment contents

1. Identification of Guizhi Fuling Pills

（1）Identification of Ramulus Cinnamomi

1）Test solution　Cut 6 g into pieces, add 50 ml of ether and heat under reflux at lower temperature for 1 hour, and filter. Evaporate the filtrate to dryness, and dissolve the residue in 1ml of ethanol as the test solution.

2) Chromatographic system and method　Apply separately 10μl of the test solution and 3 μl of the cinnamaldehyde reference solution to the silica gel G plate, and a mixture of petroleum ether (60 – 90℃) – ethyl acetate (17:3) as the mobile phase. After developing, removal of the plate, dry in air, spray with dinitrophenylhydrazine TS in ethanol. The spot in the chromatogram obtained with the test solution corresponds in the position and colour to the spot in the chromatogram obtained with the reference solution.

(2) Identification of Moutan Cortex

1) Test solution　Obtained under Identification of Cinnamomi Ramulus.

2) Chromatographic system and method　Apply separately 10μl of each of the test solution and the paeonol reference solution to the silica gel G plate, and a mixture of cyclohexane – ethyl acetate (3:1) as the mobile phase. After developing and removal of the plate, dry in air, spray with 5% ferric chloride in ethanol acidated with hydrochloric acid and heat to the spots distinct. The spot in the chromatogram obtained with the test solution corresponds in the position and colour to the spot in the chromatogram obtained with the reference solution.

(3) Identification of Paroniae Radix Rubra

1) Test solution　To the residue obtained under Identification of Cinnamomi Ramulus, add 20 ml of ethanol, ultrasonicate for 15 minutes, filter and evaporate the filtrate to dryness. Dissolve the residue in 15 ml of water, extract with two 20 ml quantities of n – butanol saturated with water. Combine the extracts, wash with water twice, each 10 ml, discard the washings, and evaporate the n – butanol extract to dryness. Dissolve the residue in 1ml of ethanol as the test solution.

2) Chromatographic system and method　Apply separately 10 μl of the test solution and 5 μl of the paeoniflorin reference solution to the silica gel G plate, and a mixture of chloroform – ethyl acetate – methanol – formic acid (40:5:10:0.2) as the mobile phase. After developing and removal of the plate, dry in air, spray with 5% vanillin in sulfuric acid and heat to the spots distinct. The blue – violet spot in the chromatogram obtained with the test solution corresponds in position to the spot in the chromatogram obtained with the reference solution.

2. Identification of Gegen Qinlian Tablets

(1) Identification of Rhizoma Coptidis

1) Test solution　To 2 tablets, pulverized to powder, add 10 ml of methanol, ultrasonicate for 15 minutes, filter, dilute 1 ml of the filtrate with methanol to 5 ml, as the test solution.

2) Reference drug solution　To 0.1 g of Coptidis Rhizoma reference drug, add 10 ml of methanol, ultrasonicate for 15 minutes, filter and use the filtrate as the reference solution.

3) Chromatographic system and method　Apply separately 1 μl each of the above two solutions and the berberine hydrochloride reference solution to the silica gel G plate, and a mix-

ture of tolune – ethyl acetate – isopropanol – methanol – concentrated ammonia TS (12 : 6 : 3 : 3 : 1) as the mobile phase. After developing in a chamber pre – equilibrated with ammonia vapour for 15 minutes and removal of the plate, dry in air, examine under ultraviolet light at 365 nm. The fluorescent spots in the chromatogram obtained with the test solution correspond in position and colour to the fluorescent spots in the chromatogram obtained with the reference drug solution and reference solution.

(2) Identification of Puerariae Lobatae Radix

1) Test solution   To 4 tablets, in fine powder, add 25 ml of ethyl acetate, ultrasonicate for 30 minutes, filter and evaporate the filtrate to dryness. Dissolve the residue in 0. 5 ml of methanol as the test solution.

2) Chromatographic system and method   Apply separately 5 μl of the test solution and 2 μl of the puerarin reference solution to the silica gel G plate, and a mixture of chloroform – methanol – water (28 : 10 : 1) as the mobile phase. After developing and removal of the plate, dry in air, expose to ammonia vapour for 15 minutes and examine under ultraviolet light at 365 nm. The fluorescent spot in the chromatogram obtained with the test solution corresponds in position and colour to the fluorescent spot in the chromatogram obtained with the reference solution.

(3) Identification of Scutellariae Radix

1) Thin layer plate   Silica gel G prepared with sodium carboxymethyl – cellulose containing 4% solution of sodium acetate (coating before experiment).

2) Test solution   To 4 tablets, in fine powder, add 30 ml of methanol, heat under reflux for 30 minutes, filter and evaporate the filtrate to dryness. Dissolve the residue in 10 ml of water, add hydrochloric acid to adjust pH to 3 – 3. 5. Extract with two 10 ml quantities of ethyl acetate, combine the extracts, evaporate to dryness, dissolve the residue in 1 ml of methanol as the test solution.

3) Chromatographic system and method   Apply separately 10μl of the test solution and 5 μl of the reference solution to the silica gel G plate containing 4% solution of sodium acetate, and a mixture of ethyl acetate – butanone – formic acid – water (5 : 3 : 1 : 1) as the mobile phase. After developing and removal of the plate, dry in air, spray with 2% ferric chloride in ethanol. The spot in the chromatogram obtained with the test solution corresponds in position and colour to the spot in the chromatogram obtained with the reference solution.

Experiment records

1. Record the TLC identification test of Guizhi Fuling Pills, plot the TLC chromatograms and calculate the R_f value of major spots.

2. Record the TLC identification test of Gegen Qinlian Tablets, plot the TLC chromatograms and calculate the R_f value of major spots.

Questions

1. To list the commonly used colouring reagents in the TLC identification. What kind of constituents can they be used to identify?

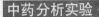

2. Why do we use ammonia vapour pre – equilibrated the chamber in identification of Rhizoma Coptidis?

3. Why do we add 4% sodium acetate to the silica gel G in identification of Radix Scitellariae?

Related materials

1. Ingredients of Guizhi Fuling Pills: Cinnamomi Ramulus 100 g, Poria 100 g, Moutan Cortex 100 g, Paeoniae Radix Rubra 100 g, Persicae Semen 100 g. Procedure: Pulverize the five ingredients to fine powder, sift, and mix well. To each 100 g of the powder add 90 – 110 g of refined honey to make to big honeyed pills. Action: To activate blood, resolve stasis and disintegrate masses. Indications: persistent abdominal masses or dysmenorrhea and eliminating mass.

2. Ingredients of Gegen Qinlian Tablets: Puerariae Lobatae Radix 1000 g, Scutellariae Radix 375 g, Coptidis Rhizoma 375 g, Glycyrrhizae Radix et Rhizoma Praeparata Cum Melle 250 g. Procedure: Pulverize 225 g of Puerariae Lobatae Radix to a fine powder. Decoct remained Puerariae Lobatae Radix and Glycyrrhizae Radix et Rhizoma Praeparata Cum Melle with water twice, 2 hours for each time. Combine the decoctions and filter, concentrate the filtrate properly. Macerate respectively Scutellariae Radix and Coptidis Rhizoma with 50% ethanol for 24 h, then percolate, and collect the solutions. Remove ethanol, combine the residues with the above concentrated solution, further concentrate to a thick extract. Add finely powdered Puerariae Lobatae Radix, mix well, dry and make granules. Dry and compressinto 1000 tablets or further coat with sugar. Action: To release the flesh, clear heat, arrest diarrhea and dysentery. Indication: Diarrhea and dysentery caused by retained dampness heat manifested as fever, vexation, thirst, foul scouring, abdominal pain and discomfort.

3. For Guizhi Fuling Pills, the volatile oil of Cinnamomi Ramulus is known to mainly contain cinnamyl aldehyde, along with cinnamyl acetate, cinnamic acid etc. The main component of Moutan Cortex is paeonol, and its derivatives, including paeonolide and paeonoside. Paeoniae Radix Rubra is known to mainly contain paeoniflorin along with oxypaeoniflorin and benzoylpaeoniflorin etc.

cinnamyl aldehyde

paeonol   paeoniflorin

4. For Gegen Qinlian Tablets, Puerariae Lobatae Radix is known to mainly contain isofla-

vonoids including puerarin and daidzin, the content of which is about 12%. Baicalin is the main component of Scutellariae Radix, the content of which is about 4% – 5%. The other flavonoids in Scutellariae Radix are wogonoside, oroxylin glucuronide etc.

puerarin   baicalin

5. The preparation of dinitrophenylhydrazine TS: Dissolve 1.5 g of 2, 4 – dinitrophenylhydrazine in 20 ml of sulfuric acid solution (1→2), dilute with water to 100 ml and filter.

实验四　附子理中丸中乌头碱及砷盐的限量检查

【目的要求】

1. 掌握用薄层色谱法对中药制剂进行限量检查的方法。

2. 熟悉砷盐检查的原理和基本操作。

【原理】

1. 乌头碱的限量检查　采用薄层色谱法，以乌头碱为对照品，供试品色谱中，在与对照品色谱相应的位置上出现的斑点应小于对照品的斑点或不出现斑点。

2. 砷盐的限量检查　金属锌与酸作用产生新生态氢与药品中的微量砷盐反应生成挥发性的砷化氢，经导气管使溴化汞试纸变色。将供试品生成的砷斑与标准砷斑比较，不得更深。反应式如下：

$$AsO_3^{3-} + 3Zn + 9H^+ \longrightarrow AsH_3 \uparrow + 3Zn^{2+} + 3H_2O$$

$$AsH_3 + 3HgBr_2 \longrightarrow 3HBr + As(HgBr)_3 (黄色)$$

$$2As(HgBr)_3 + AsH_3 \longrightarrow 3AsH(HgBr)_2 (棕色)$$

【仪器、试剂与药品】

1. 仪器　砷盐测定仪、马福炉、坩埚、微量注射器。

2. 材料　醋酸铅棉花、表面皿、漏斗、滤纸、蒸发皿、硅胶 G 板（5cm×10cm）、具塞锥形瓶、毛细管、量筒。

3. 试剂　正己烷、乙酸乙酯、二乙胺、乙醚、无水乙醇、氨试液、盐酸、氢氧化钙、溴化汞试纸、标准砷溶液（1μg/ml）、稀碘化铋钾试液、碘化钾试液、酸性氯化亚锡试液。

4. 药品　乌头碱对照品溶液（1mg/ml）、附子理中丸（市售）。

【实验内容】

1. 乌头碱的限量检查　取本品大蜜丸36g，切碎，置表面皿中，加氨试液4ml，拌匀，放置 2 小时，加乙醚 60ml，振摇 1 小时，放置 24 小时，滤过，滤液蒸干，残渣加无水乙醇 1ml 使溶解，作为供试品溶液。精密吸取供试品溶液 12μl、乌头碱对照品溶液 5μl，分别点于同一硅胶 G 薄层板上，以正己烷－乙酸乙酯－二乙胺（14:4:1）为展开剂，展开，取出，晾干，喷以稀碘化铋钾试液。供试品色谱中，在与对照品色谱相应位置上出现的斑点应小于对照品的斑点或不出现斑点。

2. 砷盐的限量检查

（1）标准砷斑的制备　精密量取标准砷溶液 2ml，置 A 瓶中（图 5－3），加盐酸 5ml 与水 21ml，再加碘化钾试液 5ml 与酸性氯化亚锡试液 5 滴，在室温放置 10 分钟后，加锌粒 2g，立即将导气管 C 与 A 瓶密塞，并将 A 瓶置 25～40℃ 水浴中反应 45 分钟，取出溴化汞试纸，即得。

（2）样品处理　取样品约 0.5g，精密称定，加等量氢氧化钙，加水少量调匀，干燥后在 500～600℃，炽灼至完全灰化，取出，放冷。

（3）检查法　将上述处理好的样品置 A 瓶中，照标准砷斑的制备，方法自"再加碘化钾试液 5ml"起，依法操作。将生成的砷斑与标准砷斑比较，不得更深。

【实验记录】

1. 绘出乌头碱限量检查的 TLC 图。
2. 记录实验过程中出现的现象和问题。
3. 计算本品中乌头碱和砷盐的限量。

【思考题】

1. 试重新设计一个乌头碱检查的实验。
2. 砷盐限量检查中加入碘化钾和氯化亚锡的目的是什么，导气管中加入醋酸铅棉花的目的是什么？

【相关资料】

1. **附子理中丸**　处方：附子（制）100g，党参 200g，白术（炒）150g，干姜 100g，甘草 100g。制法：以上五味，粉碎，过筛，混匀。每 100g 粉末用炼蜜 35～50g 加适量水泛丸，干燥，制成水蜜丸；或加炼蜜 100～120g 制成大蜜丸，即得。功能与主治：温中健脾。用于脾胃虚寒，脘腹冷痛，呕吐泄泻，手足不温。

2. **附子**　为毛茛科植物乌头 Aconitum carmichaeli Debx. 的子根的加工品。主要含有乌头碱（aconitine）、次乌头碱（hypaconitine）等生物碱，这类生物碱毒性最大。在炮制过程中乌头碱（双酯型生物碱）水解后去掉 8 位乙酰基时，其毒性为乌头碱的1/50～1/500，进一步水解失去 14 位的苯甲酸形成乌头胺，其毒性为乌头碱的1/2000～1/4000。检查附子中乌头碱的限量用于考察炮制程度，防止中毒。

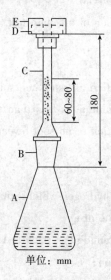

乌头碱 (aconitine)　　　　$R_1=C_2H_5$　$R_2=OH$
次乌头碱（hypaconitine）　$R_1=CH_3$　$R_2=H$

3. 砷盐限量检查装置　见图 5-3。

A. 100ml标准磨口锥形瓶
B. 中空标准磨口塞
C. 导气管（装醋酸铅棉花60mg）
D. 具孔有机玻璃旋塞
E. 中央具圆孔直径6mm的有机玻璃旋塞盖

单位：mm

图 5-3　砷盐限量检查装置

4. 导气管中装入醋酸铅棉花的作用　供试品和锌粒中可能含有少量硫化物，在酸性溶液中产生 H_2S 气体，干扰试验，故须采用醋酸铅棉花吸收除去 H_2S。

5. 碘化钾和酸性氯化亚锡作用　可用下式表示：

$$AsO_4^{3-} + 2I^- + 2H^+ \longrightarrow AsO_3^{3-} + I_2 + H_2O$$
$$AsO_4^{3-} + Sn^{2+} + 2H^+ \longrightarrow AsO_3^{3-} + Sn^{4+} + H_2O$$
$$I_2 + Sn^{2+} \longrightarrow 2I^- + Sn^{4+}$$
$$4I^- + Zn^{2+} \longrightarrow [ZnI_4]^{2-}$$
$$Sn^{2+} + Zn \longrightarrow Sn + Zn^{2+}$$

6. 试剂的配制

（1）标准砷溶液　称取三氧化二砷 0.132g，置 1000ml 量瓶中，加 20% 氢氧化钠溶液 5ml 溶解后，用适量的稀硫酸中和，再加稀硫酸 10ml，用水稀释至刻度，摇匀，作为储备液。临用前，精密量取储备液 10ml 用水稀释至刻度，摇匀，即得，每 1ml 相当于 1μg 的 As。

（2）稀碘化铋钾试液　取次硝酸铋 0.85g，加冰醋酸 10ml 与水 40ml 溶解后，即得。临用前取 5ml，加碘化钾溶液（4→10）5ml，再加冰醋酸 20ml，加水稀释至100ml，即得。

（3）酸性氯化亚锡试液　取氯化亚锡 1.5g，加水 10ml 与少量的盐酸溶解，即得。本液应临用新制。

Experiment 4　Limit Test of Aconitine and Arsenate in Fuzi Lizhong Pills

Purpose

1. To master TLC method applied in the limit test of TCM.

2. To be familiar with the principle and basic operation of arsenate test.

Principle

1. Limit test of aconitine

Use the method of thin layer chromatography, aconitine as reference substance. The size of the spot in the chromatogram obtained with the test solution is less than the corresponding spot in the chromatogram obtained with the reference solution or no spot reveals in the chromatogram obtained with the test solution.

2. Limit test of arsenate

The reaction of zinc and acid products new prepared hydrogen which can convert into volatile arsenic hydride by reaction with micro – arsentic in the drug.

Arsentic hydride can change color of the mercuric bromide test paper. Any stain produced should be no more intense than the standard stain Reaction：

$$AsO_3^{3-} + 3Zn + 9H^+ \longrightarrow AsH_3 \uparrow + 3Zn^{2+} + 3H_2O$$

$$AsH_3 + 3HgBr_2 \longrightarrow 3HBr + As(HgBr)_3 \text{（yellow）}$$

$$2As(HgBr)_3 + AsH_3 \longrightarrow 3AsH(HgBr)_2 \text{（brown）}$$

Apparatus, materials, reagents and drugs

1. Apparatus：arsenate detector, muffle furnace, xble, microsypinge.

2. Materials：lead acetate cotton wool, watch glass, funnel, filter paper, evaporating dish, silica gel G plate, cylinder.

3. Reagents：n – hexane, ethyl acetate, diethylamine, ether, dehydrated ethanol, ammonia TS, hydrochloric acid, calcium hydroxide, dilute potassium iodobismuthate TS, silver diethyldithiocarbamate, arsenic standard solution（1 μg/ml）, potassium iodide TS, acid stannous chloride TS, mercuric bromide test paper.

4. Drugs：aconitine CRS（1 mg/ml）; Fuzi Lizhong Pills（for sale）.

Experiment contents

1. Limit test of aconitine

Stir well 36 g of the big honeyed pills, cut into pieces, with 4 ml of ammonia TS in a evaporating dish, allow to stand for 2 hours, add 60 ml of ether, shake for 1 hour, stand for 24 hours, filter, evaporate the filtrate to dryness. Dissolve the residue in 1 ml of dehydrated ethanol as the test solution. Use silica gel G containing sodium carboxymethylcellulose as the coating substance and a mixture of n – hexane – ethyl acetate – diethylamine (14: 4: 1) as the moblile phase. Apply separately to the plate 12μl of the test solution and 5 μl of the aconitine solution. After developing and removal of the plate, dry it in air and spray with dilute potassium iodobismuthate TS. The size of the spot in the chromatogram obtained with the test solution is less than the corresponding spot in the chromatogram obtained with the reference solution or no spot reveals in the chromatogram obtained with the test solution.

2. Limit Test of Arsenic

(1) Preparation of arsenic standard stain   Place 2 ml of standard arsenic solution, accurately measured, add 5 ml of hydrochloric acid and 21 ml of water. Then add 5 ml of potassium iodide TS and 5 drops of acid stannous chloride TS. Allow to stand at room temperature for 10 minutes and add 2 g of zinc granules. Connect conduit C into flask A immediately (Figure 2 – 3), immerse the flask A in a water bath at 25 – 40℃ for 45 minutes. Remove the mercuric bromide test paper.

(2) Treatment of sample   To 0. 5 g, weigh accurately, add quantity of calcium hydroxide and some water, mix well. After drying, ignite in a muffle furnance at 500 – 600℃ until the incineration is complete, remove, cool.

(3) Procedure   Transfer the test preparation prepared to flask A, and proceed as described under arsenic standard stain, beginning with the words "Then add 5 ml of potassium iolide TS". Any stain produced is not more intense than the standard stain.

Experiment records

1. Draw the TLC chromatograph of limit test of aconitine.

2. Make a record of the experiment process and the problems.

3. Calculate limit of aconitine and arsenate.

Questions

1. Try to design another test of aconitine.

2. What is the purpose of adding potassium iodide TS and stannous chlorides TS and why should lead acetate cotton wool be packed into conduit in limit test for arsenic?

Related materials

1. Ingredients of Fuzi Lizhong Pills：Aconiti Lateralis Radix Preparata 100 g, Codonopsis Radix 200 g, Atractylodis Macrocephalae Rhizoma (stir – baked) 150 g, Zingibei Rhizomas 100 g, Glycyrrhizae Radix et Rhizoma 100 g. Procedure：Pulverize the above five ingredients into fine powder, sift and mix well. To each 100 g of the powder, add 35 – 50 g refined honey and a quantity of water, make water – honeyed pills and dry. Alternatively, add 100 – 120 g of refined honey to make big honeyed pills. Action：To warm the middle energizer and fortify the spleen. Indications：Spleen – stomach deficiency cold pattern, cold pain in the epigastrium, and abdomen, vomiting and diarrhea, cold limbs.

2. Prepared Common Monkshood Daughter Root is the processed daughter root of *Aconitum*

carmichaeli Debx. It's main compositions are aconitine which toxicity is the most, hypaconitine and other alkloids. The acetyl group connected to C_8 of the aconitine with double easter bonds is hydrolysed in the course of processing to form Benzoylaconitine with signal easter bond, whose toxicity is $1/50 - 1/500$ of that of the aconitine. Then the benzyl group connected to C_{14} is further hydrolysed to form aconine, whose toxicity is $1/2000 - 1/4000$ of that of aconitine. The purpose of limit test of aconitine is to inspect degree of processing and the lest toxicity.

3. Apparatus of limit test for arsenic (Figure 5 – 3).

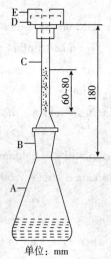

A.a 100ml conical flask with standard ground joint
B.a standard hollow ground glass stopper
C.glass conduit (a wad of lead acetate cotton wool weighing about 60mg)
D.a plastic screw (a disc of mercuric bromide test paper)
E.a plastic screw cap

单位: mm

Figure 5 – 3　Apparatus of limit test for arsonic

4. The purpose of packing lead acetate cotton wool into tube C: The minor sulfides in the sample and zinc granules could produce H_2S to interfere the test, so a wad of lead acetate cotton wool is packed into tube C to absorb H_2S.

5. The purpose of adding potassium iodide TS and stannous chloral TS can be expressed as follows:

$$AsO_4^{3-} + 3Zn + 9H^+ \longrightarrow AsO_3^{3-} + I_2 + H_2O$$
$$AsO_4^{3-} + Sn^{2+} + 2H^+ \longrightarrow AsO_3^{3-} + Sn^{4+} + H_2O$$
$$I_2 + Sn^{2+} \longrightarrow 2I^- + Sn^{4+}$$
$$4I^- + Zn^{2+} \longrightarrow [ZnI_4]^{-2}$$
$$Sn^{2+} + Zn \longrightarrow Sn + Zn^{2+}$$

6. Preparation of test solution

(1) Standard arsonic solution　Dissolve 0. 132 g of arsenic trioxide with 5 ml of 20% sodium hydroxide solution in a 1000 ml volumetric flask, neutralize with dilute sulfuric acid and add 10 ml in excess, dilute with water to volume and mix well, as a stock solution. Transfer 10 ml of the stock solution, accurately measured, to a 1000 ml volumetric flask immediately before use, add 10 ml of dilute sulfuric acid, dilute with water to volume and mix well (each ml is equivalent to 1 μg of As).

(2) Potassium iodobismuthate dilute TS　Dissolve 0. 85 g of bismuth subnitrate in a mix-

ture of 10 ml of glacial acetic acid and 40 ml of water. Before use, add 5 ml of Potassium Iodide solution (4→10) and 20 ml of glacial acetic acid to 5 ml of the solution mentioned above dilute with water to 100 ml.

(3) Stannous chloride TS Dissolve 1.5 g of stannous chloride in 10 ml of water and a small amount of hydrochloride acid. This solution should be freshly prepared.

实验五　甲苯法测定当归中的水分

【目的要求】

1. 掌握甲苯法测定中药制剂中水分的原理和操作方法。
2. 熟悉测定水分的种类及其适用范围。

【原理】

中药中水分的测定方法有烘干法、甲苯法、减压干燥法及气相色谱法，其中甲苯法适用于含挥发性成分的药品。当归中含挥发油成分，因此选用甲苯法测定其中水分的含量。

【仪器、试剂与药品】

1. **仪器**　电热套、分析天平。
2. **材料**　水分测定仪（图 5-4）、玻璃珠、长刷、铜丝、乳钵、小刀。
3. **试剂与试药**　甲苯（CP）、亚甲蓝（AR）。
4. **药品**　当归（市售品）。

【实验内容】

取本品研碎，取约 25g（相当于含水量 1~4ml），精密称定，置 A 瓶（图 5-4）中，加甲苯约 200ml，必要时加入玻璃珠数粒，将仪器各部分连接，自冷凝管顶端加入甲苯，至充满 B 管的狭细部分。将 A 瓶置电热套中或用其他适宜方法缓缓加热，待甲苯开始沸腾时，调节温度，使每秒钟馏出 2 滴。待水分完全馏出，即测定管刻度部分的水量不再增加时，将冷凝管内部先用甲苯冲洗，再用饱蘸甲苯的长刷或其他适宜的方法，将管壁上附着的甲苯推下，继续蒸馏 5 分钟，放冷至室温，拆卸装置，如有水黏附在 B 管的管壁上，可用蘸甲苯的铜丝推下，放置，使水分与甲苯完全分离（可加亚甲蓝粉末少量，使水染成蓝色，以便分离观察）。检读水量，并计算供试品中的含水量（%）。

【实验记录】

1. 记录实验原始数据。
2. 计算供试品中的含水量。

【思考题】

1. 实验中所用仪器是否要烘干？为什么？
2. 为什么说本法适用于含挥发性成分的中药制剂中水分的测定？

【相关资料】

1. 当归中主要成分 当归中主要含有挥发性物质如藁本内酯、有机酸如阿魏酸等。功能与主治：补血活血，调经止痛，润肠通便。用于血虚萎黄，眩晕心悸，月经不调，经闭痛经，虚寒腹痛，风湿痹痛，跌扑损伤，痈疽疮疡，肠燥便秘。酒当归活血通经。用于经闭痛经，风湿痹痛，跌扑损伤。

2. 水分测定法 烘干法适用于不含或少含挥发性成分的药品，主要是将药品在 100～105℃ 干燥 5～6 小时，使其完全失去水分（两次干燥后减重不超过 5mg），根据干燥前后减失的重量来计算含水量。甲苯法适用于含挥发油成分的药品。减压干燥法适用于含有挥发性成分的贵重药品，主要是在常温低压条件下，使样品中的水分蒸发并被干燥剂（五氧化二磷）吸收，再利用重量差异计算含水量，此法不破坏药品及药品中的挥发性成分。

甲苯法水分测定装置见图 5-4，包括 500ml 短颈圆底烧瓶（A）、水分测定管（B）、直形冷凝管（C，外管长 40cm）。

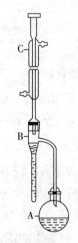

图 5-4 甲苯法水分测定装置

3. 注意事项 实验要用化学纯甲苯直接测定，必要时甲苯可先加水少量，充分振摇后放置，将水层分离弃去，经蒸馏后使用。样品应先粉碎成直径不超过 3mm 的颗粒。用减压干燥法测定水分时，样品应过 2 号筛。

Experiment 5 Determination of Water in Angelica Sinensis Radix

Purpose

1. To master the principle and operational method of water determination in Traditional Chinese Medicine by toluene distillation method.

2. To be familiar with different methods of water determination and the relevant suitable range.

Principle

To determinate water, four methods can be chosen: drying in oven method, toluene distillation method, drying under reduced pressure method and gas chromatographic method. Toluene distillation method is used for the determination of water in drugs containing volatile constituents. There are volatile constituents in Angelica Sinensis Radix, so toluene distillation method is used to determinate water content.

Apparatus, Materials and Reagents

1. Apparatus: band heater, analytical balance.

2. Materials: apparatus for determination of water by toluene distillation method (Figure 5 – 4), bead, brush, copper wire, mortar, knife.

3. Reagents: toluene (CP), methylene blue (AR).

4. Drugs: Tongxuan Lifei Pills (for sale).

Experiment contents

Place 25 g of triturated Tongxuan Lifei pills which is anticipated to yield about 1 – 4 ml of water and accurately weighed, in the flask A (Figure 5 – 4), add about 200 ml of toluene and a few glass beads if necessary. Assemble the apparatus and fill the receiving tube B with toluene through the condenser. Heat the flask gently, when toluene begins to boil, adjust the temperature and allow to distill at a rate of 2 drops per second. When the volume of water in the receiving tube does not increase any more, rinse the inside of condenser with toluene and push down the toluene adhering to the wall with a brush or other suitable tools. Continue the distillation for 5 minutes, cool to room temperature and disconnect the apparatus. Push down any droplet of water adhering to the wall of the receiving tube with a copper wire wetted with toluene. Allow to stand until water is completely separated from toluene in the receiving tube (a small amount of methylene blue may be added to facilitate observation). Record the volume of water distilled and calculate the percentage of water in Tongxuan Lifei Pills (%).

Experiment records

1. Record original data of the experiment.

2. Calculate the content of water in Tongxuan Lifei Pills.

Questions

1. Whether all parts of the apparatus used in the experiment need to be dried in an oven? Why?

2. Why toluene distillation method is suitable to determinate water content in Traditional Chinese Medicine Preparation containing volatile constituents?

Related materials

1. Constituents in Angelicae Sinensis Radix: Angelicase Sinensis Radix mainly contains volatile constituent such as ligustilide and organic acids such as ferulic acid, etc. Action: To nourish blood, activate blood, regulate menstruation, relieve pain, moisten the intestines and relax the bowels. Indications: Blood deficiency with sallow complexion, dizziness, palpitations, menstrual irregularities, amenorrhea and dysmenorrhea, deficiency cold abdominal pain, painful bi disorder caused by wind – dampness, traumatic injuries, abscesses and cellulitis, sore and ulcer, and constipation caused by intestinal dryness. Angelicae Sinensis Radix (processed with wine) could activate blood and unblock the meridian, and could be used for amenorrhea and dysmenorrhea, painful bi disorder caused by wind – dampness, and traumatic injuries.

2. In the four methods, drying in oven method is used for the determination of water in drugs containing no or scarcely any volatile constituents, the main operation is drying drugs in an oven at 100 – 105 ℃ for 5 – 6 hours, repeating the operation until the water is completely evaporated and the difference between two successive weighing is not more than 5 mg. Calculate the percentage content of water in the substance being examined according to the weight loss on drying. Toluene distillation method is used for the determination of water in drugs containing volatile constituents. Drying under reduced pressure method is used for determination of water in noble drugs containing volatile constituents, the method is to evaporate water in the substance being examined in the condition of normal temperature and reduced pressure, and then water being evaporated is absorbed by dryer (phosphorous pentoxide) , and calculate the percentage content of water in the substance being examined according to the weight loss on drying, the method does not destroy the substance being examined as well as the volatile constituents in it.

Apparatus for determination of water by toluene distillation method (Figure 5 – 4) consist of a 500 ml round bottom flask (A) , a graduated receiving tube (B) and a reflux condenser (C) (approximately 40 cm in length) .

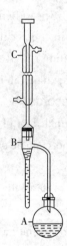

3. The experiment should use chemically pure toluene directly to determinate water, and toluene used in this procedure should be saturated with water and distilled if necessary. The substance being examined is usually broken into granules or pieces with less than 3 mm in diameter. The substance being examined using the drying under reduced pressure method has to pass through a No. 2 sieve.

Figure 5 – 4　Apparatus for determination of water by toluene distillation method

实验六　气相色谱法测定藿香正气水中乙醇的含量

【目的要求】

1. 掌握气相色谱法测定中药制剂中乙醇含量的方法。

2. 熟悉气相色谱定量分析操作方法。

【原理】

利用气相色谱法测定成药在 20℃时乙醇的含量（%，V/V），并用内标法计算含量。

【仪器、试剂与药品】

1. **仪器** 气相色谱仪（FID 检测器）、微量进样器。
2. **材料** 量瓶（100ml）、移液管、具塞锥形瓶（25ml）。
3. **试剂** 无水乙醇，正丙醇。
4. **药品** 藿香正气水（市售品）。

【实验内容】

1. 色谱条件与系统适用性试验 色谱柱为填充柱或毛细管柱，以直径为 0.25 ~ 0.18mm 的二乙烯苯 - 乙基乙烯苯型高分子多孔小球作为载体；柱温为 120 ~ 150℃；载气为 N_2；FID 检测器。理论板数按正丙醇峰计算应不低于 700，乙醇和正丙醇两峰的分离度应大于 2。

2. 校正因子测定

（1）对照溶液配制 精密量取恒温至 20℃的无水乙醇 4ml、5ml、6ml，分别置 100ml 量瓶中，分别精密加入恒温至 20℃的正丙醇（内标物）5ml，加水稀释至刻度，混匀，即得，作为对照溶液。

（2）测定校正因子 取上述 3 种对照溶液各 2μl，注入气相色谱仪，分别连续进样 5 次，测定峰面积，按下式计算校正因子。

$$校正因子（f） = \frac{A_S/c_S}{A_R/c_R}$$

式中，A_S——内标物质正丙醇的峰面积；

A_R——对照品无水乙醇的峰面积；

c_S——内标物质正丙醇的浓度；

c_R——对照品无水乙醇的浓度。

3. 供试品溶液的制备 精密量取恒温至 20℃的藿香正气水 10ml 和正丙醇 5ml，加水稀释成 100ml，混匀，即得。

4. 测定法 吸取供试品溶液 2μl，连续进样 3 次，记录供试品中待测组分乙醇和内标物质正丙醇的峰面积，按下式计算含量：

$$含量（c_X） = f \times \frac{A_X}{A_S/c_S}$$

式中，A_X——乙醇的峰面积；

c_X——乙醇的浓度；

A_S——内标物质正丙醇的峰面积；

c_S——内标物质正丙醇的浓度。

【实验记录】

记录实验数据，计算乙醇含量。

【思考题】

1. 内标物应符合哪些条件？

2. 中药制剂中哪些剂型需要检查乙醇含量？

【相关资料】

1. **藿香正气水** 处方：苍术160g，陈皮160g，厚朴（姜制）160g，白芷240g，茯苓240g，大腹皮240g，生半夏160g，甘草浸膏20g，广藿香油1.6ml，紫苏叶油0.8ml。制法：以上十味，苍术、陈皮、厚朴、白芷分别用60%乙醇作溶剂，浸渍24小时后进行渗漉，前三种各收集初漉液400ml，后一种收集初漉液500ml，备用，继续渗漉，收集续漉液，浓缩后并入初漉液中。茯苓加水煮沸后，80℃温浸两次，第一次3小时，第二次2小时，取汁；生半夏用冷水浸泡，每8小时换水一次，泡至透心后，另加干姜13.5g，加水煎煮二次，第一次3小时，第二次2小时；大腹皮加水煎煮3小时，甘草浸膏打碎后水煮化开；合并上述水煎液，滤过，滤液浓缩至适量，广藿香油、紫苏叶油用乙醇适量溶解。合并以上溶液，混匀，用乙醇与水适量调整乙醇含量，并使全量成2050ml，静置，滤过，灌装，即得。功能与主治：解表化湿，理气和中。用于外感风寒、内伤湿滞或夏伤暑湿所致的感冒，症见头痛昏重、胸膈痞闷、脘腹胀痛、呕吐泄泻；胃肠型感冒见上述证候者。

2. **制备过程中所用溶剂为乙醇** 成药中含乙醇量的高低对于成药有效成分的含量、所含杂质的量和类型以及制剂的稳定性等都有影响，所以《中国药典》规定对该类制剂需做乙醇量检查。

Experiment 6　Determination of Ethanol in Huoxiang Zhengqi Tincture by GC

Purpose

1. To master the method of determination of ethanol in Traditional Chinese Medicine Preparation by gas chromatography.

2. To be familiar with the operational method of GC.

Principle

GC is used to determine the content of ethanol (%, V/V) of patent medicine under 20℃ and calculate the content of ethanol by internal standard method.

Apparatus, materials, reagents and drugs

1. Apparatus：gas chromatogram（FID detector），microsyringe.

2. Materials：graduated cylinder（100 ml），transfer pipette，stopper conical flask（25 ml）.

3. Reagents：dehydrated ethanol，n - Propanol.

4. Drugs: Huoxiang Zhengqi Tincture (for sale).

Experiment contents

1. Chromatographic system and system suitability

Column: capillary column or packed column, using porous polymer beads of ethyl vinyl-benzene cross – linked with divinylbenzene 0. 25 – 0. 18 mm in diameter as support; column temperature: 120 – 150 ℃; carrier gas: Nitrogen; Flame Ionization Detector. The number of theoretical plates of the column is not less than 700, calculated with the reference of the peak of n – propanol, the resolution of the peaks of ethanol and n – propanol is more than 2.

2. Determination of correction factor

(1) Preparation of reference solutions   Measure accurately 4 ml, 5 ml, 6 ml of dehydrated ethanol warmed to 20 ℃ under constant temperature to 100 ml volumetric flasks separately, add 5 ml of n – propanol (internal standard substance) warmed to 20 ℃ under constant temperature respectively, dilute with water to volume, mix well as the reference solutions.

(2) Determination of correction factor   Carry out 5 replicate injections for each of the three reference solutions mentioned above. Inject accurately 2 μl each of the above three reference solutions into the column separately, determine the peak areas, calculate the correct factor using the following equation.

$$\text{Correction factor } (f) = A_S c_R / A_R c_S$$

A_S——peak area of the internal standard substance n – propanol;

A_R——peak area of the reference preparation ethanol;

c_S——concentration of the internal standard substance n – propanol;

c_R——concentration of the reference preparation ethanol.

3. Preparation of test solution

Transfer accurately 10 ml of Huoxiang Zhengqi Tincture and 5 ml of n – propanol, which are warmed to 20 ℃ under constant temperature, to 100 ml volumetric flasks, dilute with water to volume, mix well as the test solution.

4. Assay

Inject 2 μl of the test solution into column, carry out successively 3 injections, record the peak areas of the ethanol and the internal standard substance n – propanol in the test solution, calculate the content as follows:

$$\text{Content } (c_X) = f \times A_X \times c_S / A_S$$

A_X——peak area of ethanol;

c_X——concentration of ethanol;

A_S——peak area of the internal standard substance n – propanol;

c_S——concentration of the internal standard substance n – propanol.

Experiment record

Record the assay data and calculate the content of ethanol.

Questions

1. What conditions should internal standard substance comply with?

2. Which kinds of preperation require determination of ethanol?

Related materials

1. Ingredients of Huoxiang Zhengqi Tincture: Atractylodis Rhizoma 160 g, Citri Reticulatae Pericarpium 160 g, Magnoliae Officinalis Cortex (processed with ginger) 160 g, Angelicae Dahuricae Radix 240 g, Poria 240 g, Arecae Pericarpium 240 g, Pinelliae Rhizoma 160 g, Glycyrrhizae Extractum 20 g, Pogostermonis Oil 1. 6 ml, Perillae Folii Oil 0. 8 ml. Procedure: Macerate separately Atractylodis Rhizoma, Citri Reticulatae Pericarpium for 24 hours, using 60% ethanol as solvent. Percolate, collect 400 ml of the initial percolate of the former three drugs and 500 ml of the later for latter use. Collect the successive percolate, concentrate, and combine with the initial percolate respectively. Boil Poria with water, macetate at 80 ℃ for two times, 3 hours and 2 hours respectively and combine the decoctions; macerate Pinelliae Rhizoma with cold water, change water every 8 hours until softened thoroughly, add 13. 5 g of dried ginger, decoct with water for two times, 3 hours and 2 hours respectively; decoct Arecae Pericarpium with water for 3 hours, pulverize and dissolve Glycyrrhizae Extractum with water on boiling; combine the above decoctions, filter, concentrate the filtrate properly. Dissolve Pogostemonis Oil and Perillae Folii Oil in a quantity of ethanol. Combine the above solutions, mix well; adjust the ethanol content with ethanol and water, make up the total volume to 2050 ml, allow to stand, filter, and pack. Action: To release the exterior pattern, resolve dampness, regulate qi and harmonize the middle. Indications: Cold caused by external contracted wind – cold, internal dampness stagnation or summer dampness, manifested as headache, dizziness, heavy sensation, stuffiness and oppression in the chest and the hypochondrium, distending pain in the stomach and abdomen, vomiting, diarrhea; gastrointestinal flu with the pattern mentioned above.

2. Huoxiang Zhengqi Tincture use ethanol as solvent during preparation. As the content of ethanol influences the content of effective components, the pattern of impurity contained and suitability of preparation in traditional Chinese patent medicine, *Pharmacopoeia of the people's Republic of China* describes the content of ethanol must be determined in these preparations.

实验七 黄连上清丸中重金属的检查

【目的要求】

1. 掌握中药制剂炽灼的基本操作方法。

2. 熟悉中药制剂经消化后进行重金属检查的方法与原理。

【原理】

中药制剂常含有大量的有机化合物，在进行重金属检查前必须先进行有机破坏，再与硫代乙酰胺或硫化钠反应，生成黑色硫化物混浊。采用目视比色法观察比较样品与标准品溶液的颜色深浅，判断样品所含重金属是否超标。

【仪器、试剂与药品】

1. **仪器**　电炉、马福炉、坩埚、分析天平、恒温水浴锅、干燥器。

2. **材料**　25ml 纳氏比色管及比色管架、移液管、量瓶（25ml）、烧杯、量筒、蒸发皿、乳钵、小刀。

3. **试剂与试药**　重蒸水、硫酸（AR）、硝酸、盐酸、酚酞指示剂、醋酸盐缓冲液（pH 3.5）、标准铅溶液（10μg/ml）、氨试液、硫代乙酰胺试液。

4. **药品**　黄连上清丸（市售品）。

【实验内容】

1. **供试品溶液的制备**　取本品水丸或水蜜丸 15g，研碎，或取大蜜丸 30g，剪碎，过二号筛，取约 1.0g，精密称定，置已炽灼至恒重的坩埚中，精密称定，缓缓炽灼至完全炭化（或在电炉上缓缓加热至冒白烟，但不得起明火），放冷至室温，加硫酸 0.5～1ml 使湿润，低温加热至硫酸蒸气除尽后，再在马福炉中 500～600℃炽灼使完全灰化，移置干燥器中，放冷至室温，精密称定后，再在 500～600℃炽灼至恒重，放冷，加硝酸 0.5ml，蒸干，至氧化氮蒸气除尽后，放冷，加盐酸 2ml，置水浴锅上蒸干后，加水 15ml，滴加氨试液至对酚酞指示剂显中性，再加醋酸盐缓冲液（pH 3.5）2ml，微热溶解后，完全转移至纳氏比色管中，加水稀释成 25ml。

2. **对照品溶液的制备**　取配制供试品溶液的试剂，置蒸发皿中蒸干后，加醋酸盐缓冲液（pH 3.5）2ml 与水 15ml，微热溶解后，移至纳氏比色管中，加标准铅溶液 2.5ml，再用水稀释成 25ml。

3. **测定法**　在样品与对照品纳氏比色管中分别加硫代乙酰胺试液 2ml，摇匀，放置 2 分钟，同置白纸上，自上向下透视，样品管中颜色与对照品管比较，不得更深。

【实验记录】

1. 记录实验原始数据及实验结果。

2. 记录实验中出现的问题并说明原因。

【思考题】

1. 根据实验计算黄连上清丸的重金属含量限度。

2. 制备对照品溶液时，为什么要取制备供试品溶液的试剂？

【相关资料】

1. **黄连上清丸**　处方：黄连 10g，栀子（姜制）80g，连翘 80g，蔓荆子（炒）80g，防风 40g，荆芥穗 80g，白芷 80g，黄芩 80g，菊花 160g，薄荷 40g，大黄（酒炙）320g，黄柏（酒炒）40g，桔梗 80g，川芎 40g，石膏 40g，旋覆花 20g，甘草 40g。制法：以上十七味，粉碎成细粉，过筛，混匀。用水泛丸，干燥，制成水丸；或每 100g

粉末用炼蜜 30~40g 加适量的水泛丸，干燥，制成水蜜丸；或每 100g 粉末加炼蜜150~170g 制成大蜜丸，即得。功能与主治：散风清热，泻火止痛。用于风热上攻、肺胃热盛所致的头晕目眩、暴发火眼、牙齿疼痛、口舌生疮、咽喉肿痛、耳痛耳鸣、大便秘结、小便短赤。

2. **重金属检查的方法**　在对中药制剂中的有机化合物进行有机破坏时，炽灼温度对重金属的影响很大，温度越高重金属损失越多。《中国药典》规定炽灼温度应控制在 500~600℃，以使其完全灰化。炽灼残渣加 0.5ml 硝酸加热处理，使消化完全，必须蒸干除尽氧化氮，蒸干后加盐酸使成盐酸盐，水浴加热蒸干，赶除残留盐酸，加水溶解，调 pH 3.5，依法检查。

重金属在实验条件下都能与硫代乙酰胺或硫化钠反应显色，生成黑色硫化物混浊，再采用目视比色法观察比较样品与对照品溶液的颜色深浅，判断样品所含重金属是否超标。标准铅溶液常以 Pb^{2+} 为代表，其原理为：

在酸性溶液中

$$CH_3CSNH_2 + H_2O \longrightarrow CH_3CONH_2 + H_2S \uparrow$$
$$Pb^{2+} + H_2S \longrightarrow PbS \downarrow （黑色）$$

在碱性溶液中

$$Pb^{2+} + Na_2S \longrightarrow PbS \downarrow （黑色） + 2Na^+$$

3. **试剂的配制**

（1）标准铅溶液　称取硝酸铅 0.160g，置 1000ml 量瓶中，加硝酸 5ml 与水 50ml 溶解后，用水稀释至刻度，摇匀，作为贮备液。临用前，精密量取贮备液 10ml，置 100ml 量瓶中，加水稀释至刻度，摇匀，即得（每 1ml 相当于 10μg 的 Pb）。配制与贮存用的玻璃容器均不得含铅。

（2）酚酞指示剂　取酚酞 1g，加乙醇 100ml 使溶解，即得。

（3）醋酸盐缓冲液（pH 3.5）　取无水氯化钠 20g，加水 300ml 溶解后，加溴酚蓝指示液 1ml 及冰醋酸 60~80ml，至溶液从蓝色转变为纯绿色，再加水稀释至 1000ml，即得。

（4）氨试液　取浓氨溶液 400ml，加水使成 1000ml，即得。

（5）硫代乙酰胺试液　取硫代乙酰胺 4g，加水使溶解成 100ml，置冰箱中保存。临用前取混合液（由 1mol/L 氢氧化钠溶液 15ml、水 5.0ml 及甘油 20ml 组成）5.0ml，加上述硫代乙酰胺溶液 1.0ml，置水浴上加热 20 秒钟，冷却，立即使用。

4. **注意事项**　实验中对马福炉的使用要严格按操作规程操作；对照品溶液的配制应从"加硝酸 0.5ml，蒸干"开始。

Experiment 7　Test of Heavy Metals in Huanglian Shangqing Pills

Purpose

1. To master the basic operational method of ignition of Traditional Chinese Medicine Preparation.

2. To be familiar with the test method and principle of heavy metals in Traditional Chinese

Medicine Preparation after being nitrated.

Principle

Traditional Chinese Medicine Preparation always contains large number of organic compound, so it must be destructed organically before testing the heavy metals, and then reacts with thioacetamide TS or sodium sulfide TS to produce black turbidity. Compare the colour of the sample with that of the standard solution using method of colourimetry by visual observation to judge whether the heavy metals content of the sample is overrun.

Apparatus, materials, reagents and drugs

1. Apparatus: electric cooker, Muffle furnace, crucible, analytical balance, water bath, desiccator.

2. Materials: Nessler cylinders (25 ml), shelf, transfer pipette, volumetric flask (25 ml), beaker, measuring cylinder, evaporating dish, mortar, knife.

3. Reagents: redistilled water, sulfuric acid (AR), nitric acid, hydrochloric acid, phenolphthalein IS, salt acetate BS (pH 3.5), standard lead solution (10 μg/ml), ammonia TS, thioacetamide TS.

4. Drugs: Huanglian Shangqing Pills (for sale).

Experiment contents

1. Preparation of test solution

Cut 15 g of water pills or water – honeyed pills or 30 g of big honeyed pills in pieces, pass through a No. 2 sieve. Place accurately weighed 1.0 g of sample being examined in a suitable crucible previously ignited to constant weight. Weigh accurately, heat gently until it is thoroughly charred (or heat gently on the electric cooker until white fumes appear but no obvious fire built), cools to room temperature and moisten the residue with 0.5 – 1 ml of sulfuric acid. Heat gently until white fumes are no longer evolved and then ignite at 500 ~ 600 ℃ until the incineration is complete. Cool in a desiccator and weigh accurately, ignite again at 500 – 600 ℃ to constant weight. Add 0.5 ml of nitric acid, evaporate to dryness, heat until nitrous oxide fumes are no longer evolved. Cool, add 2 ml of hydrochloric acid, evaporate to dryness on a water bath, add 15 ml of water, followed by ammonia TS dropwise until the solution is neutral to phenolphthalein IS, then add 2 ml of acetate BS (pH 3.5) and warm to effect dissolution. Transfer the resulting solution to Nessler cylinder B, dilute with water to 25 ml.

2. Preparation of reference solution

Place the same quantity of the same reagents used for the preparation of test solution in a porcelain dish and evaporate to dryness, heat gently and dissolve in 2 ml of acetate BS (pH 3.5) and 15 ml of water, transfer to the Nessler cylinder A and add 2.5 ml of standard lead solution, dilute with water to 25 ml.

3. Procedure

To each cylinder add 2 ml of thioacetamide TS and mix well, allow to stand for 2 minutes, compare the colour produced by viewing down the vertical axis of the cylinders against a white

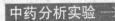

background. The colour produced in cylinder of sample (cylinder B) is not more intense than that produced in cylinder of the standard (cylinder A).

Experiment records

1. Record original data of the experiment and calculate the experimental result.

2. Make a record of the problems appeared during the experiment and illuminate the causes of the problems.

Questions

1. Calculate content limit of heavy metals in Huanglian Shangqing Pills according to the experiment?

2. Why take the same quantity of the same reagents used for the preparation of test solution in preparation of reference solution?

Related materials

1. Ingredients of Huanglian Shangqing Pills: Coptidis Rhizoma 10 g, Gardeniae Fructus (processed with ginger) 80 g, Forsythiae Fructus 80 g, Viticis Fructus (stir – baked) 80 g, Saposhnikoviae Radix 40 g, Schizonepetae Spica 80 g, Angelicae Dahuricae Radix 80 g, Scutellariae Radix 80 g, Chrysanthemi Flos 160 g, Menthae Herba 40 g, Rhei Radix et Rhizoma (stir – baked with wine) 320 g, Phellodendri Cortex (stir – baked with wine) 40 g, Platycodonis Radix 80 g, a Chuanxiong Rhizom 40 g, Gypsum Fibrosum 40 g, Inulae Flos 20 g, Glycyrrhizae Radix et Rhizoma 40 g. Procedure: Pulverize the above seventeen ingredients to fine powder, sift and mix well. Make water pills and dry; To each 100 g of the powder, add 30 – 40 g of refined honey and a quantity of water to make water – honeyed pills and dry; To each 100 g of the powder, add 150 – 170 g of refined honey to make big honeyed pills. Action: To dissipate wind – heat, purge fire and relieve pain. Indications: Dizziness and vertigo, epidemic conjunctivitis, toothache, mouth and tongue sores, swollen sore throat, swollen sore throat, ear pain and tinnitus, constipation, short voiding of dark urine caused by wind – heat upside, exuberant heat of lung and stomach.

2. The test method of heavy metals: In the procedure of organic compound destruction, the ignition temperature has great effect on heavy metals, the higher the temperature is, the more heavy metals lose. It is prescribed in Chinese pharmacopoeia that the ignition temperature should be controlled at 500 – 600℃ to make the incineration complete. Add 0.5 ml of nitric acid to the residue on ignition and heat to make it nitrified thoroughly, evaporate to dryness until nitrous oxide fumes are no longer evolved, add hydrochloric acid to produce hydrochloric salt, evaporate to dryness on a water bath, add water to dissolve it, adjust pH value to 3.5 and determinate according to the given method.

Heavy metals can react with thioacetamide TS or sodium sulfide TS to produce blackprecipitate in experimental condition. And then compare the colour of the sample with that of the standard solution using method of colourimetry by visual observation to judge whether the heavy metals content of the sample is overrun. Pb^{2+} can be a normal representation of the standard solution, the principles are as follows:

In acidic solution:

$$CH_3CSNH_2 + H_2O \longrightarrow CH_3CONH_2 + H_2S \uparrow$$

$$Pb^{2+} + H_2S \longrightarrow PbS \downarrow \text{ (black)}$$

In alkaline solution:

$$Pb^{2+} + Na_2S \longrightarrow PbS \downarrow \text{ (black)} + 2Na^+$$

3. The preparation of reagents

(1) Standard lead solution Dissolve 0.160 g of lead nitrate with 5 ml of nitric acid and 50 ml of water in a 1000 ml volumetric flask, dilute to volume with water, mix well (stock solution). Transfer 10 ml of the stock solution, accurately measured, into a 100 ml volumetric flask, dilute with water to volume and mix well (each ml is equivalent to 10 μg of Pb). This solution should be prepared immediately before use. All glassware used for the preparation and preservation of standard lead solution should be free from lead.

(2) Phenolphthalein IS Dissolve 1 g of phenolphthalein in 100 ml of ethanol.

(3) Salt acetate BS (pH 3.5) Dissolve 20 g of anhydrous sodium acetate in 300 ml of water, add 1 ml of bromophenol blue TS and 60 – 80 ml of glacial acetic acid until the colour changes from blue to pure green, and then dilute with water to 100 ml.

(4) Ammonia TS Dilute 400 ml of concentrated ammonia solution with water to 1000 ml.

(5) Thioacetamide TS Dissolve 4 g of the thioacetamide in water to make 100 ml. Store in refrigerator. Add 1.0 ml of thioacetamide solution to 5.0 ml of mixture consisting of 15 ml sodium hydroxide solution (1 mol/L), 5.0 ml of water and 20 ml of glycerin before use, heat for 20 seconds in water bath, cool and use immediately.

4. The use of Muffle furnace must follow the operating regulation strictly. The preparation of reference solution should be carried out from "add 0.5 ml of nitric acid and evaporate to dry".

实验八 灯盏细辛注射液的有关物质检查

【目的要求】

1. 掌握注射剂杂质检查的目的、原理及操作方法。

2. 熟悉草酸盐检查的原理和基本操作。

【原理】

注射剂有关物质检查项目主要包括：蛋白质检查（加磺基水杨酸或鞣酸检查）、鞣质检查（加鸡蛋清或明胶氯化钠试液检查）、重金属检查（照中国药典方法检查，不得超过百万分之十）、砷盐检查（照中国药典方法检查，不得超过百万分之二）、草酸盐检查（加氯化钙检查）、钾离子检查（加四苯硼酸钠检查）、树脂检查（加盐酸或冰醋酸检查）。

【仪器、试剂及药品】

1. **仪器** 超声波清洗器、紫外灯、马福炉；

2. **材料** 漏斗、分液漏斗、纳氏比色管、试管、滤纸；

3. **试剂** 冰醋酸、三氯甲烷、蒸馏水、10%硫酸乙醇溶液、鞣酸试液、稀醋酸、氯化钠明胶试液、盐酸、稀氢氧化钠、3%氯化钙溶液、酚酞指示液、标准钾离子溶液、标准砷溶液、标准铅溶液、碱性甲醛溶液、3%乙二胺四醋酸二钠溶液、3%四苯硼钠溶液、三乙胺；

4. **药品** 灯盏细辛注射液（市售品）。

【实验内容】

1. **蛋白质** 取本品1ml，置试管中，滴加鞣酸试液1~3滴，不得产生浑浊。

2. **鞣质** 取本品1ml，置试管中，加稀醋酸1滴，再加氯化钠明胶试液4~5滴，不得出现浑浊或沉淀。

3. **树脂** 取本品5ml，置分液漏斗中，加三氯甲烷10ml振摇提取，分取三氯甲烷液，置水浴上蒸干，残渣加冰醋酸2ml使溶解，置具塞试管中，加水3ml，混匀，放置30分钟，应无絮状物析出。

4. **草酸盐** 取本品10ml，用稀盐酸调pH 1~2，滤过，滤液通过聚酰胺柱（100~200 内径为1cm，干法装柱），收集初流出液2ml，调pH 5~6，加3%氯化钙溶液2~3滴，放置10分钟，不得出现浑浊或沉淀。

5. **钾离子** 取本品10ml，蒸干，先用小火炽灼至炭化，再在500~600℃炽灼至完全灰化，加稀醋酸使溶解，置25ml量瓶中，加水稀释至刻度，混匀，作为供试品溶液。取10ml纳氏比色管两支，甲管中精密加入标准钾离子溶液0.8ml，加碱性甲醛溶液（取甲醛溶液，用0.1mol/L氢氧化钠调节pH至8.0~9.0）12滴、3%乙二胺四醋酸二钠溶液2滴、3%四苯硼钠溶液0.5ml，加水稀释成10ml。乙管中精密加入供试品溶液1ml，与甲管同时依法操作，摇匀。甲、乙两管同置黑纸上，自上向下透视，乙管中显出的浊度与甲管比较，不得更浓。

【实验记录】

1. 记录实验过程中出现的现象和问题。

2. 记录灯盏细辛注射液的检查实验结果。

【思考题】

注射剂中杂质检查项目主要有哪些。

【相关资料】

1. **灯盏细辛注射液的处方** 灯盏细辛800g。制法：略。功能与主治：活血祛瘀，通络止痛。用于瘀血阻滞，中风偏瘫，肢体麻木，口眼歪斜，言语謇涩及胸痹心痛；缺血性中风、冠心病心绞痛见上述证候者。

2. 试剂的配制

（1）鞣酸试液：取鞣酸 1g，加乙醇 1ml，加水溶解并稀释至 100ml，即得。本液应临用新制。

（2）氯化钠明胶试液：取白明胶 1g 与氯化钠 10g，加水 100ml，置不超过 60℃ 的水浴上微热使溶解。本液应临用新制。

（3）酚酞指示液：取酚酞 1g，加乙醇 100ml，使溶解，即得。变色范围 8.3～10（无色～红色）

（4）醋酸盐缓冲液（pH 3.5）：取醋酸铵 25g，加水 25ml 溶解后，加 7mol/L 盐酸溶液 38ml，用 2mol/L 盐酸溶液或 5mol/L 氨溶液准确调 pH 至 3.5（电位法指示），用水稀释至 1000ml，即得。

（5）标准钾离子溶液：取硫酸钾适量，研细，于 110℃ 干燥至恒重，精密称取 2.330g，置 1000ml 量瓶中，加水适量使溶解并稀释至刻度，摇匀，作为贮备液。临用前，精密量取贮备液 10ml，置 100ml 量瓶中，加水稀释至刻度，摇匀，即得。（每 1ml 相当于 100μg 的钾）。

（6）碱性甲醛溶液：取甲醛溶液，用 0.1mol/L 氢氧化钠调节 pH 至 8.0～9.0。

（7）3% 四苯硼钠溶液：取四苯硼钠 31g，加水 215ml 使溶解加入新配制的氢氧化铝凝胶（取三氯化铝 4.0g，溶于 100ml 水中，在不断搅拌下缓缓滴加氢氧化钠试剂至 pH 8～9），加氯化钠 71.1g，充分摇匀。加水 250ml，振摇 15min，静置 10min，滤过，滤液中滴加氢氧化钠试剂至 pH 8～9，再加水稀释至 1000ml，摇匀。

Experiment 8 Limit Test for Related Substances of Dengzhanxixin Injection

Purpose

1. To master the purpose and principle and operational method in the test for foreign matter of injection.

2. To be familiar with the principle and basic operation of oxalate test.

Principle

The test items of foreign matter about injection mainly include: the test for protein (the test of adding tannic acid), tannin (the test of adding albumen or sodium chloride and galatin TS), the limit test for heavy metals (the test of complying with the method in Chinese Pharmacopoeia, not more than 0.001%), the limit test for arsenic (the test of complying with the method in Chinese Pharmacopoeia, not more than 0.0002%), the test for oxalate (the test of adding calcium chloride), the test for potassium iron (test by sodium tetraphenylborate), the test for resin (the test of adding hydrochloric acid or glacial acetic acid).

Apparatus, materials, reagents and drugs

1. Apparatus: ultrasonic surge, muffle furnace;

2. Materials: Nessler cylinder, test tube, filter paper, funnel, separate funnel;

3. Reagents: glacial acetic acid, chloroform, distilled water, 10% sulfuric acid in ethanol solution, tannic acid TS, dilute acetic acid, sodium chloride and galatin TS, hydrochloric acid, dilute sodium hydroxide, 3% calcium chloride solution, phenolphthalein IS, acetate BS (pH 3.5), potassium iron standard solution, standard arsenic solution, standard lead solution, alkaline formaldehyde, 3% disodium edetate solution, 3% sodium tetraphenylborate solution, triethylamine;

4. Drugs: Dengzhanxixin injection (for sale).

Experiment contents

1. **Protein** Transfer 1ml into a test tube, add 1 ~ 3 drops of tannic acid TS, no opalescence is produced.

2. **Tannin** Transfer 1ml into a test tube, add 1 drop of dilute acetic acid, then add 4 ~ 5 drops of sodium chloride and galatin TS, no opalescence or precipitate is produced.

3. **Resin** Take 5ml into a transfer it into a separating funnel, add 10 ml of chloroform, shake well, separate the chloroform solution, evaporate on a water bath to dry, add 2 ml of glacial acetic acid in the residue to dissolve it, then pour into a test tube with plug, add 3 ml of water and mix well, allow to stand for 30 minutes, no flocculus should appear.

4. **Oxalate** Transfer 10ml into a test tube, adjust to pH 1 ~ 2 with dilute hydrochloric acid, then filter, the filtrate is subjected to a polyamide column (100 ~ 200 mesh size, 1 g, column internal diameter 1 cm, dry packing), collect the eluent 2ml, adjust the filtrate to pH 5 ~ 6, add 2 ~ 3 drops of 3% calcium chloride solution, allow to stand for 10 minutes, no opalescence or precipitate is produced.

5. **Potassium iron** Take 10 ml and evaporate, ignite till carbonized with weak flame, then incinerate at 500 ~ 600℃ until carbon – free, add dilute acetic acid to dissolve, and transfer into 25 ml volumetric flask, dilute with water to the volume and mix well, use as a test solution. Take two Nessler cylinder, measure accurately potassium iron standard solution 0.8 ml in tube A, add 12 drops of alkaline formaldehyde (measure formaldehyde solution, adjust the pH value to 8.0 ~ 9.0 with sodium hydroxide), 2 drops of 3% disodium edetate solution, 0.5 ml of 3% sodium tetraphenylborate solution, dilute with water to 10 ml. Measure accurately 1 ml of the test solution in tube B, process as what done on tube A at the same time, shake well. Compare to opalescence produced by viewing down the vertical axis of the cylinders against a black background, opalescence of tube B should not be heavier than that of tube A.

Experiment records

1. Make a record of the experiment process and the problems.

2. Record the test of foreign matter.

Questions

What are the main test items of foreign matter about injection?

Related materials

1. **Ingredients of Dengzhanxixin Injection**: Erigerontis Herba 800 g. Procedure: Omit-

ted. Action：To activate blood, dispel stasis, unblock the collateral, and relieve pain. Indications：Static blood obstruction, wind – stroke, hemiplegia, numbness of limbs, deviated eyes and mouth, dysphasia, chest bi disorder, and heart pain；Ischemic stroke, and angina pectoris of coronary heart disease with the symptoms described above.

2. The preparation of reagents：

（1）Tannic acid TS：Dissolve 1 g of tannic acid in 1 ml of alcohol and dilute with water to 100 ml. This solution should be freshly prepared.

（2）Sodium chloride and galatin TS：Dissolve 1 g of gelatin and 10 g of sodium chloride in 100 ml of water by heat on a water bath at a temperature below 60 ℃.

（3）Phenolphthalein IS：Dissolve 1 g of phenolphthalein in 100 ml of ethanol. Colour changes from colourless to red（pH 8. 3 ~ 10. 0）.

（4）Acetate BS（pH 3. 5）：Dissolve 25 g of ammonium acetate in 25 ml of water, add 38 ml of hydrochloric acid solution（7 mol/L）. Adopt the potentiometric acid solution（2 mol/L）or ammonia solution（5 mol/L）and dilute with water to 1000 ml.

（5）Potassium iron standard solution：Place suitable potassium sulfate, grind into fine power, dry to constant weigh at 110℃, weigh 2. 330 g accurately, put into 1000 ml volumetric flask, add sufficient water to dissolve and dilute to the volume, shake well, use as store solution. Immediately before using, measure accurately the store solution 10 ml in 100 ml volumetric flask, dilute with water to volume and shake well（each ml equals to 100 μg of potassium）.

（6）Alkaline formaldehyde：Measure formaldehyde solution, adjust the pH value to 8. 0 ~ 9. 0 with sodium hydroxide.

（7）3% sodiumtetraphenylborate solution：Dissolve 31 g of sodium tetraphenylborate in 215 ml of water with shake. Add freshly prepared aluminum hydroxide gel（dissolve 4. 0 g of aluminum chloride in 100 ml of water, add sodium hydroxide TS dropwise with stirring until the pH is 8 – 9）, 71. 1 g of sodium chloride and stir thoroughly. Add 250 ml of water and shake for 15 minutes, allow to stand for 10 minutes and filter. Add sodium hydroxide TS dropwise to the filtrate until the pH is 8 – 9, and then dilute with water to 1000 ml, mix well.

实验九　酸性染料比色法测定华山参片总生物碱的含量

【目的要求】

1. 掌握酸性染料比色法的基本原理及操作方法。
2. 了解分光光度法在中药制剂含量测定中的应用及测定结果的意义。

【原理】

利用生物碱类药物（B），在适当 pH 介质中，可与氢离子（H^+）结合成阳离子（BH^+），而一些酸性染料如溴百里酚蓝、溴酚蓝、溴甲酚紫、溴甲酚绿等，可解离成阴离子（In^-），上述阳离子与阴离子定量地结合成有机络合物（$BH^+ In^-$），即离子对。该离子对可定量地用有机溶剂提取，在一定波长处测定该有色离子对溶液的吸收度，即可计算出生物碱的含量，其反应式为：

$$BH^+ + In^- \longrightarrow (BH^+ In^-)_{水相} \longrightarrow (BH^+ In^-)_{有机相}$$

【仪器、试剂与药品】

1. **仪器**　可见 – 紫外分光光度计、超声波清洗器、恒温水浴锅。

2. **材料**　量瓶（25ml）、移液管、分液漏斗、具塞锥形瓶（25ml）、定量滤纸。

3. **试剂**　枸橼酸 – 磷酸氢二钠缓冲液（pH 4.0）、0.04% 溴甲酚绿溶液（用上述缓冲液配制）、三氯甲烷。

4. **药品**　硫酸阿托品（$C_{17}H_{23}NO_3$）$_2 \cdot H_2SO_4 \cdot H_2O$（中国食品药品检定研究院）；华山参片（市售品）。

【实验内容】

1. 对照品溶液的制备　取在 120℃ 干燥至恒重的硫酸阿托品，精密称定，加水制成每 1ml 相当于含莨菪碱 7μg 的溶液，即得。

2. 供试品溶液的制备　取本品 40 片，除去糖衣，精密称定，研细，精密称取适量（约相当于 12 片重量），置具塞锥形瓶内，精密加入枸橼酸 – 磷酸氢二钠缓冲液（pH 4.0）25ml，振摇 5 分钟，放置过夜，用干燥滤纸滤过，弃去初滤液，取续滤液，即得。

3. 测定法　精密量取供试品溶液与对照品溶液各 2ml，分别置分液漏斗中，各精密加枸橼酸 – 磷酸氢二钠缓冲液（pH 4.0）10ml，再精密加入 0.04% 溴甲酚绿溶液 2ml，摇匀，用 10ml 三氯甲烷振摇提取 5 分钟，待溶液完全分层后，分取三氯甲烷液，用三氯甲烷湿润的滤纸滤入 25ml 量瓶中，再用三氯甲烷提取 3 次，每次 5ml，依次滤入量瓶中，并用三氯甲烷洗涤滤纸，滤入量瓶中，加三氯甲烷至刻度，摇匀。

分别在 415nm 波长处测定吸光度，计算，即得。本品含生物碱以莨菪碱（$C_{17}H_{23}NO_3$）计，应为标示量的 80.0% ~ 120%。

【实验记录】

记录实验数据，计算总生物碱的含量。

【思考题】

1. 采用本方法所测定的总生物碱含量是相对含量还是绝对含量？说明结果的意义。

2. 影响本实验含量测定准确性的因素有哪些？

【相关资料】

1. 华山参片由华山参浸膏制成。制法：取华山参，粉碎成粗粉，用含 0.1% 盐酸的乙醇作溶剂，浸渍 24 小时，进行渗漉，至漉液色淡为止，漉液减压浓缩至稠膏状，测定生物碱含量，加辅料适量，制成颗粒，压片，包糖衣，即得。功能与主治：温肺平喘，止咳祛痰。用于寒痰停饮犯肺所致的气喘咳嗽、吐痰清稀；慢性气管炎、喘息性气管炎见上述证候者。

2. 华山参为茄科植物 *Physochlaina infundibulris* Kuang 的干燥根，含多种莨菪烷类生物碱，如 l – 莨菪碱（l – hyoscyamine，阿托品为莨菪碱的消旋体，pK_a = 9.65）、东莨菪碱（scopolamine，pK_a = 6.20）、山莨菪碱（anisodamine）等。

3. 水相 pH 的选择：含一个碱性基团的生物碱，形成 1∶1 的离子对，最好在 pH 5.2 ~ 6.4 时提取；而含二个碱性基团的二元生物碱形成 1∶2 的离子对，为使第二个碱基团成盐，则最好在较低的 pH 3.0 ~ 5.8 时提取。

4. 枸橼酸 – 磷酸氢二钠缓冲液（pH 4.0）的配制。甲液：取枸橼酸 21g，或无水枸橼酸 19.2g，加水使溶解成 1000ml，置冰箱内保存。乙液：取磷酸氢二钠 71.63g，加水溶解成 1000ml。取上述甲液 61.45ml 与乙液 38.55ml，混合，摇匀即得。

Experiment 9   Determination of the Total Alkaloids in Tabellae Physochlainae by Acid – dye Colorimetry

Purpose

1. To master the principle and the method of acid – dye colorimetry.

2. To be acquainted with the application of spectrophotometry in the assay of Traditional Chinese Medicine Preparation and significance of the results.

Principle

In certain pH value, the alkaloids (B) and the hydrogen ion (H^+) combine into the cation (BH^+). Meanwhile, some acid – dyes, for example, bromothymol blue, bromophenol blue, bromocresol purple, bromocresol green etc., turn into the anion (In^-). The above two kinds of ions can combine into the colored compound ($BH^+ In^-$), which can be extracted by organic solvent quantitatively. Then assay the absorbance of the compound at a certain wavelength, calculate the content of alkaloids. The equation is：

$$BH^+ + In^- \longrightarrow (BH^+ In^-)_{aqueous\ phase} \longrightarrow (BH^+ In^-)_{organic\ phase}$$

Apparatus, materials, reagents and drugs

1. Apparatus：ultraviolate – visible spectrophotometer, ultrasonic surge, water bath.

2. Materials：volumetric flasks (25 ml), transfer pipettes, separate funnel, stopper conical flasks (25 ml), quantitative filter paper.

3. Reagents：citric acid – sodium dihydrogen phosphate BS (pH 4.0), 0.04% bromocresol green solution (prepared with above BS), chloroform.

4. Drugs: atropine sulfate CRS [($C_{17}H_{23}NO_3$) · H_2SO_4 · H_2O] ; Tabellae Physochlain-ae (for sale) .

Experiment contents

1. Preparation of reference solution

Weigh accurately a quantity of atropine sulfate CRS, dried to constant weight at 120 ℃, dissolve in water to produce a solution containing 7 μg per ml of hyoscyamine as the reference solution.

2. Preparation of test solution

Weigh accurately 40 tablets, remove sugar coats, and pulverize to fine powder. Weigh accurately a quantity of the powder (equivalent to about 12 tablets) in a stopper conical flask, add accurately 25 ml of citric acid – sodium dihydrogen phosphate BS (pH 4. 0), shake for 5 minutes, and allow to stand for overnight. Filter with dry filter paper, discard the initial filtrate and use the successive filtrate as the test solution.

3. Assay

Measure accurately 2 ml each of the reference solution and the test solution in separators, add accurately 10 ml of citric acid – sodium dihydrogen phosphate BS (pH 4. 0) and 2 ml of 0. 04% bromocresol green solution prepared with above BS respectively, and shake well, extract with 10 ml of chloroform for 5 minutes by shaking, separate the chloroform layer and filter with filter paper moisten with chloroform, in 25 ml volumetric flasks. Continue to extract the aqueous layer with three 5 ml quantities of chloroform and filter to the flask, wash the filter paper with chloroform and filter to the flask, dilute with chloroform to the volume, shake well.

Carry out the method for spectrophotometry, measure separately the absorbance at the wavelength of 415 nm and calculate the content accordingly. It contains not less than 80. 0% and not more than 120% of the labeled amount of the alkaloids, calculated as hyoscyamine ($C_{17}H_{23}NO_3$) .

Experiment record

Record the assay data and calculate the content of the total alkaloids.

Questions

1. Is the total alkaloids content determined in this experiment relative content or absolute content? Instruct the significance of the results.

2. Which factors would influence the accuracy of the assay in this experiment?

Related materials

1. Tabellae Physochlainae is made up of Radix Physochlainae extract. Procedure: Pulverize the Radix Physochlainae to coarse powder, using ethanol containing 0. 1% of hydrochloric acid as the solvent, macerate for 24 hours, then percolate until the colour of percolated solution is pale, concentrated the solution in vacuum to thick extract, determine the content of alkaloids, to the extract add a quantity of excipients, make granules, compress into tablets and coat with sugar. Action: To warm the lung and calm panting, suppress cough and dispel phlegm. Indications: Wheezing and cough, expectoration of clear thin sputum caused by cold

– phlegm and retained fluid invading the lung; chronic tracheitis and asthmatic tracheitis with the pattern mentioned above.

2. Radix Physochlainae is from the roots of *Physochlaina infundibulris* Kuang, alkaloids are its main components, including l – hyoscyamine (atropine is its racemic, pK_a = 9.65), scopolamine (pK_a = 6.20), and anisodamine.

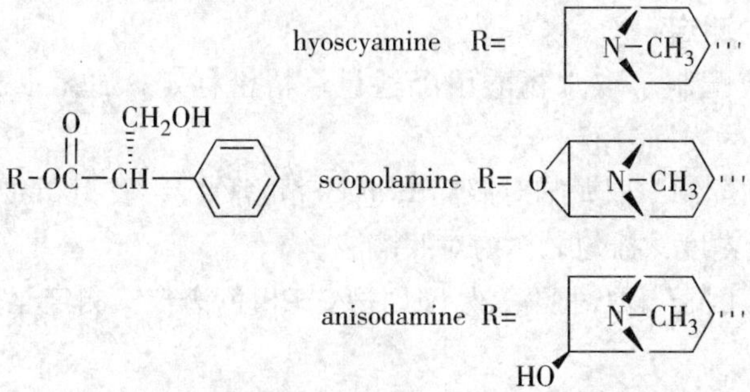

hyoscyamine R=

scopolamine R=

anisodamine R=

3. The pH value of aqueous phase: The pH value of aqueous phase should be adjusted to pH 5.2 ~ 6.4 if the alkloids are all monoatomic base, in which the alkaloid cation (BH^+) and the acid – dye anion (In^-) combine in a ratio of 1:1. While for those alkaloids belonging to bi-atomic base, the pH value of aqueous phase should be adjusted to pH 3.0 – 5.8 in order that the second basic group is also combined by the acid – dye anion.

4. The preparation of citric acid – sodium dihydrogen phosphate BS (pH 4.0).

(1) Dissolve 21 g of citric acid or 19.2 g of anhydrous citric acid in water to make 1000 ml, preserve in a refrigerator.

(2) Dissolve 71.63 g of disodium hytrogen phosphate in water to make 1000 ml.

Take 61.45 ml of solution (a) and 38.55 ml of solution (b) and mix well.

实验十　气相色谱法测定西瓜霜润喉片中冰片的含量

【目的要求】

1. 掌握气相色谱法测定中药制剂中成分含量的方法和原理。

2. 熟悉气相色谱仪进行含量测定的操作过程。

【原理】

利用中药制剂所含有效成分具挥发性，可用气相色谱法对其进行含量测定，因成药中所有组分不能全部出峰，故采用内标法定量。

【仪器、试剂与药品】

1. **仪器**　气相色谱仪（FID 检测器）、超声波清洗器、微量进样器。

2. **材料**　量瓶（100ml）、移液管、具塞锥形瓶（25ml）。

3. **试剂**　无水乙醇。

4. **药品**　水杨酸甲酯，龙脑对照品（中国食品药品检定研究院）；西瓜霜润喉片

（市售品）。

【实验内容】

1. 色谱条件与系统适用性试验 色谱柱为改性聚乙二醇–20M 毛细管柱（柱长 30m，内径 0.53mm，膜厚度 1.2μm）；柱温为 135℃；载气为 N_2，柱前压 100kPa 左右；氢气（H_2）50kPa；空气 50kPa；FID 检测器。理论板数按龙脑峰计算应不低于 8000。

2. 校正因子的测定

（1）内标溶液配制 取水杨酸甲酯适量，精密称定，加无水乙醇制成每 1ml 含 0.2mg 的溶液，作为内标溶液。

（2）对照溶液配制 取龙脑对照品 15mg，精密称定，置 100ml 量瓶中，加入内标溶液溶解并稀释至刻度，摇匀，作为对照溶液。

（3）测定校正因子 取对照溶液 1μl 注入气相色谱仪，测定至少 5 次，按下式计算校正因子。

$$校正因子（f）=\frac{A_S/c_S}{A_R/c_R}$$

式中，A_S——内标物质水杨酸甲酯的峰面积；

A_R——对照品龙脑的峰面积；

c_S——内标物质水杨酸甲酯的浓度；

c_R——对照品龙脑的浓度。

3. 供试品溶液的制备 取重量差异项下的本品，研细，取约 1.5g，精密称定，置具塞锥形瓶中，精密加入内标溶液 5ml，密塞，摇匀，称定重量，超声处理（功率 250W，频率 50kHz）20 分钟，放冷，再称定重量，用无水乙醇补足减失的重量，摇匀，静置沉降（或离心），上清液作为供试品溶液。

4. 测定法 吸取供试品溶液 1μl，注入气相色谱仪，连续进样 3 次，记录供试品中待测组分龙脑和内标物质水杨酸甲酯的峰面积，按下式计算含量：

$$含量（c_X）=f\times\frac{A_X}{A_S/c_S}$$

式中，A_X——龙脑的峰面积；

c_X——龙脑的浓度；

A_S——内标物质水杨酸甲酯的峰面积；

c_S——内标物质水杨酸甲酯的浓度。

【实验记录】

记录实验数据，计算冰片的含量。

【思考题】

1. 气相色谱仪常用的检测器有几种？说明各自的特点。

2. 中药制剂中哪些成分可以用气相色谱法分析？

【相关资料】

1. 西瓜霜润喉片 处方：西瓜霜，冰片，薄荷素油，薄荷脑。制法：以上四味，西瓜霜粉碎成细粉，加入蔗糖粉、糊精，取枸橼酸及胭脂红适量，加水溶解，与上述粉末混匀，制成颗粒，干燥，加入薄荷素油、薄荷脑、冰片及橘子香精适量，混匀，密闭，压制成片，即得。功能与主治：清音利咽，消肿止痛。用于防治咽喉肿痛，声音嘶哑，喉痹，喉痛，喉蛾，口糜，口舌生疮，牙痛；急、慢性咽喉炎，急性扁桃体炎，口腔溃疡，口腔炎，牙龈肿痛。

2. **冰片** 是西瓜霜润喉片的主要成分，为合成产品，主要含龙脑和异龙脑峰。

龙脑（*l*-borneol）　　　　　　异龙脑（*d*-borneol）

3. **注意事项** 实验前，必须对气相色谱仪整个气路系统进行检漏。如有漏气，及时处理。开机前先通气，实验结束，先关机，后关气。由于样品中挥发性成分较多，样品干燥时，要注意方法和温度。

Experiment 10　Determination of Borneolum Syntheticum in Xiguashuang Runhou Tablets by GC

Purpose

1. To master the method and principle of determining the content of components in Traditional Chinese Medicine Preparation by gas chromatography.

2. To be familiar with the operational process of determining the content with gas chromatography.

Principle

Gas chromatography is used to determine the content of components being of volatility in traditional Chinese patent medicine. Since not all components in the patent can output peaks in chromatogram, the content is determined by the internal standard method.

Apparatus, materials, reagents and drugs

1. Apparatus: GC chromatogram (FID detector), ultrasonic surge, microsyringe.

2. Materials: volumetric flask (100 ml), transfer pipette, stopper conical flask (25 ml).

3. Reagents: dehydrated ethanol.

4. Drugs: methyl salicylate, (±) – borneol CRS (provided by National Institute for Food and Drug Control); Xiguashuang Runhou Tablets (for sale).

Experiment contents

1. Chromatographic system and system suitability

Chromatographic column is the modified polyethyleneglycol – 20 M capillary column (column length 30 m, inner diameter 0.53 mm, film thickness 1.2 μm); column temperature is 135 ℃; carrier gas is N_2, column front pressure 100 kPa or so, H_2 50 kPa; air 50 kPa; FID detector. The number of theoretical plates of the column is not less than 8000, calculated with reference to the peak of ($\pm$) – borneol.

2. Determination of correction factor

(1) Preparation of internal standard solution　Dissolve a quantity of methyl salicylate, accurately weighed, in dehydrated ethanol to produce a solution containing 0. 2 mg per ml as the internal standard solution.

(2) Preparation of reference solution　Dissolve 15 mg of ($\pm$) – borneol CRS, accurately weighed, in a 100 ml volumetric flask and dilute with the internal standard solution to volume, mix well as the reference solution.

(3) Determination of correction factor　Inject accurately 1 μl of reference solution into the gas chromatograph, determine 5 times at least, calculate the correction factor as follows:

$$\text{Correction factor } (f) = A_S c_R / A_R c_S$$

A_S——peak area of the internal standard substance (methyl salicylate) ;

A_R——peak area of the reference substance [($\pm$) – borneol] ;

c_S——concentration of the internal standard substance (methyl salicylate) ;

c_R——concentration of the reference substance [($\pm$) – borneol] .

3. Preparation of test solution

Pulverize the tablets obtained under the test of weigh variation to fine powder, weigh accurately 1. 5 g to a stopper conical flask, add accurately 5 ml of the internal standard solution, mix thoroughly and weigh. Ultrasonicate for 20 minutes (power 250 W, frequency 50 kHz), stand to cool, weigh again, replenish the lost weight with dehydrated ethanol, mix well, allow subside (or centrifuge), use the supernatant as the test solution.

4. Assay

Inject 1 μl of the test solution into the column, continually inject 3 times, record the peak areas of the test component [($\pm$) – borneol] and the internal standard substance (methyl salicylate) in the test solution, calculate the content as follows:

$$\text{Content } (c_X) = f \times A_X c_S / A_S$$

A_X——peak area of [($\pm$) – borneol] ;

c_X——concentration of [($\pm$) – borneol] ;

A_S——peak area of the internal standard substance (methyl salicylate) ;

c_S——concentration of the internal standard substance (methyl salicylate) .

Experiment record

Record the assay data and calculate the content of ($\pm$) – borneol.

Questions

1. What kinds of detectors are commonly used in gas chromatogram, and describe their characteristics?

2. Please list the components in traditional Chinese patent medicines that can be analyzed by GC.

Related materials

1. Ingredients of Xiguashuang Runhou Tablets：Mirabilitum Praeparatum, Borneolum Syntheticum, Peppermint Oil（Oleum Menthae Dementholatum）, Mentholum. Procedure：Pulverze Mirabilitum Praeparatum to fine powder, add a quantity of sucrose powder and dextrin, dissolve a quantity of citric acid and carmine in water, mix thoroughly with the above powder, make granules, dry, add Peppermint Oil, Mentholum and a quantity of orange essence, mix thoroughly, close tightly, compress into tablets. Action：To clear the voice and soothe the throat, disperse swelling and relieve pain. Indications：Prevention of swollen sore throat, hoarseness of voice, throat impediment, tonsillitis, oral erosion, mouth and tongue sores, gum abscess；acute and chronic pharynx golaryngitis, mouth ulcers, stomatitis and swelling painful gums.

2. Borneolum Syntheticum, which is the mixture of borneol and isoborneol, is the main component of Xiguashuang Runhou Tablets.

3. Before experiment, check the system of gas flow, examine if there are any leaks. First aerate, then power the GC equipment, and reverse the order when experiment finish. As the sample contain a lot of volatile components, be careful for the method and temperature of desiccation.

实验十一　HPLC 法测定银杏叶片中总黄酮醇苷的含量

【目的要求】

1. 掌握高效液相色谱法及其在中药制剂有效成分含量测定中的应用。
2. 熟悉高效液相色谱法的操作步骤。

【原理】

银杏叶片为银杏叶提取物制得，主要成分为黄酮醇苷，黄酮醇苷可酸水解成黄酮醇类化合物。因此，本实验利用高效液相色谱法，以槲皮素、山奈素、异鼠李素为对照，在 360nm 波长处测定银杏叶片中总黄酮醇苷的含量。

【仪器、试剂与药品】

1. **仪器**　高效液相色谱仪、微量进样器、分析天平、超声波清洗器、恒温水浴锅。
2. **材料**　具塞锥形瓶、移液管、滤纸、漏斗、冷凝管（24#）、圆底烧瓶（24#，100ml）、量瓶（50ml）、微孔滤膜。
3. **试剂与试药**　甲醇（色谱纯）、重蒸水、磷酸（分析纯）、25% 盐酸溶液。
4. **药品**　槲皮素对照品、山奈素对照品、异鼠李素对照品（中国食品药品检定研究院）；银杏叶片（市售品）。

【实验内容】

1. **色谱条件与系统适用性试验**　以十八烷基硅烷键合硅胶为填充剂；甲醇－0.4% 磷酸溶液（50∶50）为流动相，检测波长为 360nm。理论板数按槲皮素峰计算应不低于 2500。

2. 对照品溶液的制备　分别取槲皮素、山柰素、异鼠李素对照品适量，精密称定，加甲醇制成每 1ml 含 30μg、30μg、20μg 的混合溶液，作为对照品溶液。

3. 供试品溶液的制备　取本品 10 片，除去包衣，精密称定，研细，取约相当于总黄酮醇苷 19.2mg 的粉末，精密称定，置具塞锥形瓶中，精密加入甲醇 20ml，密塞，称定重量，超声处理 20 分钟（功率 250W，频率 33kHz），放冷，再称定重量，用甲醇补足减失的重量，摇匀，滤过，精密量取续滤液 10ml，置 100ml 圆底烧瓶中，加甲醇10ml、25% 盐酸溶液 5ml，摇匀，置水浴中加热回流 30 分钟，迅速冷却至室温，转移至 50ml 量瓶中，用甲醇稀释至刻度，摇匀，滤过，取续滤液，即得。

4. 测定法　分别精密吸取对照品溶液与供试品溶液各 10μl，注入液相色谱仪，测定，分别计算槲皮素、山柰素、异鼠李素的含量，按下式换算成总黄酮醇苷的含量。

总黄酮醇苷 = （槲皮素含量 + 山柰素含量 + 异鼠李素含量）×2.51

本品每片含总黄酮醇苷规格（1）不得少于 9.6mg，规格（2）不得少于 19.2mg。

【实验记录】

1. 记录实验原始数据及相关色谱图。
2. 记录实验过程中出现的现象和问题。
3. 计算本品中总黄酮醇苷的含量。

【思考题】

1. 用超声提取法提取总黄酮醇苷有哪些优点？
2. 实验中影响含量测定结果的因素有哪些？怎样使测定结果更准确？

【相关资料】

1. **银杏叶片**　处方：银杏叶提取物 40g［规格（1）］或 80g［规格（2）］，加辅料适量，制成颗粒，压制成 1000 片，包糖衣或薄膜衣，即得。功能与主治：活血化瘀通络。用于瘀血阻络引起的胸痹心痛、中风、半身不遂、舌强语謇；冠心病稳定型心绞痛、脑梗死见上述证候者。

2. **银杏叶**　为银杏科植物银杏 *Ginkgo biloba* L. 的干燥叶，主要含银杏双黄酮、芸香苷等黄酮类成分及二萜内酯类成分，如银杏内酯 A、银杏内酯 B 以及银杏内酯 C 等。以上两类成分为银杏叶制剂中的主要有效成分，为治疗心脑血管疾病的有效药物。

3. **黄酮醇苷**　可酸水解成黄酮醇类化合物，主要是槲皮素、山柰素、异鼠李素等，其结构式如下。

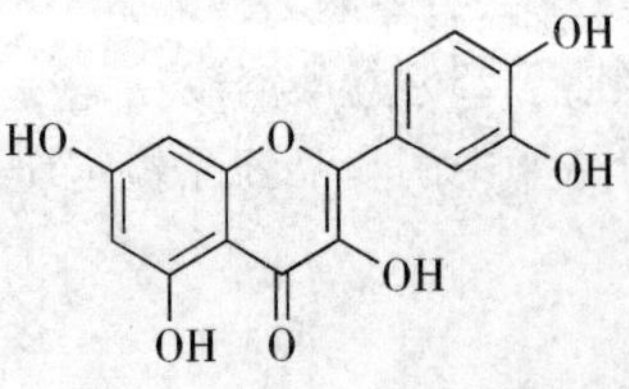

槲皮素 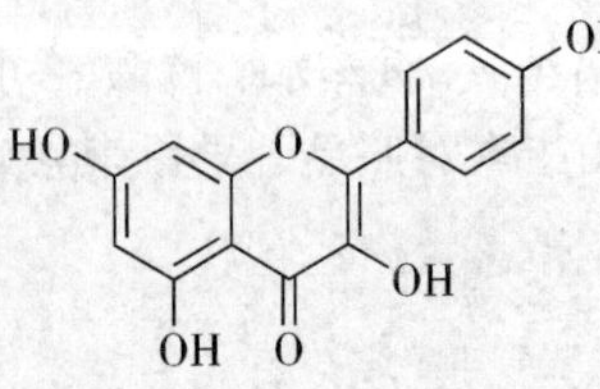　　　　　　　　　山柰素 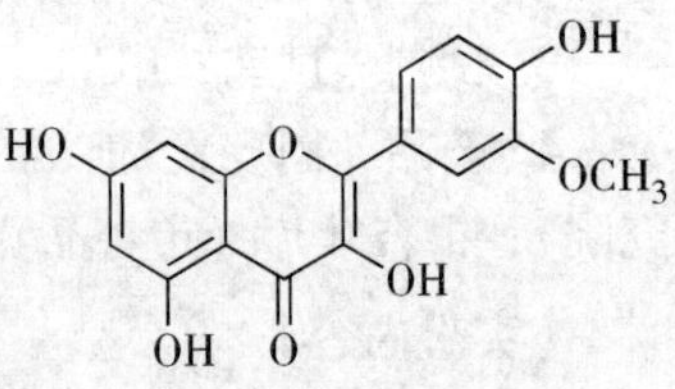　　　　　　　　　异鼠李素

Experiment 11　　Determination of Total Amount of Flavonol

Glycosides in Yinxingye Tablets by HPLC

Purpose

1. To master the application of HPLC in assay of effective ingredients of Traditional Chinese patent medicine.

2. To be acquainted with the method for the determination of total composition in patents.

Principle

Yinxingye Tablet is made from the extract of Folium Ginkgo, and its main components are flavonol glycosides which can produce flavonols by acid hydrolysis. This experiment determines total amount of flavonol glycosides by HPLC at 360 nm and quercetin, kaempferol, and isorhamnetin are used as reference.

Apparatus, materials, reagents and drugs

1. Apparatus: HPLC, microsyringe, analytical balance, ultrasonic surge, water bath.

2. Materials: stopper conical flask, transfer pipette, filter paper, funnel, condenser pipe ($24^{\#}$), round bottom flask ($24^{\#}$, 100 ml), volumetric flask (50 ml), micro – porous filtration membrane.

3. Reagents: methanol (chromatographically pure), re – distilled water, phosphoric acid (AR), 25% hydrochloric acid TS.

4. Drugs: quercetin CRS, kaempferol CRS, isorhamnetin CRS (provided by National Institute Food and Drug control); Yinxingye Tablets (for sale).

Experiment contents

1. Chromatographic system and system suitability

Use octadecylsilane bonded silica gel as the stationary phase and a mixture of methanol – 0.4% solution of phosphoric acid (50:50) as the mobile phase. As detector a spectrophotomrter set at 360 nm. The number of theoretical plates of the column is not less than 2500, calculated with the reference to the peak of quercetin.

2. Preparation of reference solution

Dissolve quercetin CRS, kaempferol CRS, isorhamnetin CRS, add methanol in methanol to prepare a mixed solution respectively containing 30 μg, 30 μg, 20 μg per ml respectively as the reference solutions.

3. Preparation of test solution

Weigh accurately 10 tablets, remove sugar coats, pulverize to fine powder. Weigh accurately the powder, equal to about 19.2 mg of total flavonoid glycosides, to a stopper conical flask, add accurately 20 ml of methanol, stopper tightly, weigh and ultrasonicate (power, 250W; frequency, 33 kHz) for 20 minutes, allow to cool, weigh again, replenish the lost weight with methanol, mix well, filter and transfer accurately 10 ml of successive filtrate into a 100 ml round bottom flask. Add 10 ml of methanol and 5 ml of 25% hydrochloric acid TS, shake well, heat under reflux for 30 minutes, cool quickly to ambient temperature, transfer accurately to a 50 ml volumetric flask, add methanol to volume, and shake well, filter and use the successive filtrate as the test solution.

4. Assay

Accurately inject 10 μl each of the reference solution and the test solution respectively, into the column and determine the contents of three flavonoids respectively. Calculate the content of total amount of flavonol glycosides using the following equation.

The content of total amount of flavonol glycosides = (the content of quercetin + the content of kaempferol + the content of isorhamnetin) ×2.51.

It contains not less than 9.6 mg in specification (1) and not less than 19.2 mg in specification (2) of total amount of flavonol glycosides per tablet.

Experiment records

1. Record original data and relative chromatogram of the experiment.

2. Record the experiment process and the problems.

3. Calculate the content of total flavonol glycosides in the sample.

Questions

1. What are the advantages of ultrasonic extraction of flavonol glycosides?

2. What are the factors affecting the result of the assay? How to improve the accuracy of the result?

Related materials

1. Ingredients and procedure of Yinxingye Tablets: Add 40 g [specification (1)] or 80 g [specification (2)] of Ginkgo Leaves extract and a quantity of excipients, mix thoroughly, make granules, dry, compress into 1000 tablets and coat with sugar or film. Acton: To active blood, resolve stasis and unblock the collaterals. Indications: Chest impediment and heart a pain, wide - stroke, hemiplegia, sluggish tongue caused by stable angina due to coronary heart disease, cerebrovascular block with the pattern mentioned above.

2. Gingkgo leaf is the dried leaf of *Gingkgo biloba* L. (Ginkgoaceae). It mainly contains flavonol glycosides, e. g. ginkgetin, rutin and diterpenoid lactone, such as ginkgolides A, B, C. These above are the effective compounds to treat heart and brain blood vessel disease.

3. Quercetin, kaempferol and isorhamnetin are all flavonols produced from flavonol glycosides by acid hydrolysis, the chemical structure of them are as follows:

quercetin   kaempferol   isorhamnetin

实验十二　注射用益气复脉（冻干）的 HPLC 指纹图谱

【目的要求】

1. 掌握 HPLC 指纹图谱法在中药注射剂质量控制中的应用。
2. 熟悉 HPLC 指纹图谱方法的建立。

【原理】

采用高效液相色谱法，建立多批注射用益气复脉冻干粉针的指纹图谱，并采用相似度评价软件对所建立的指纹图谱进行评价，确定参比峰，计算各共有指纹峰的相对保留时间及相对峰面积。

【仪器、试剂与药品】

1. **仪器**　高效液相色谱仪、微量进样器。
2. **材料**　量瓶（10ml）、微孔滤膜。
3. **试剂**　乙腈（色谱纯）、重蒸水、磷酸（分析纯）、甲醇（分析纯）。
4. **药品**　对照品人参皂苷 Re、Rg$_1$ 及人参二醇、人参三醇、五味子醇甲、五味子甲素、五味子乙素；注射用益气复脉冻干粉针（市售品）。

【实验内容】

1. **色谱条件与系统适用性试验**　以十八烷基硅烷键合硅胶为填充剂；乙腈 – 0.05% 磷酸溶液为流动相进行梯度洗脱（表 5 – 1），检测波长为 203nm。理论板数按人参皂苷 Rg$_1$ 峰计算应不低于 2000。

表 5 – 1　液相梯度洗脱条件

时间（分钟）	A 0.05% 磷酸	B 乙腈
0 ~ 10	80→70	20→30
10 ~ 18	70→69	30→31
18 ~ 30	69→67	31→33
30 ~ 40	67→55	33→45
40 ~ 50	55→45	45→55
50 ~ 70	45→10	55→90

2. **对照品溶液的制备**　取人参皂苷 Re、Rg$_1$、人参二醇、人参三醇、五味子醇甲、五味子甲素、五味子乙素对照品适量，精密称定，用甲醇溶解，分别制备成一定浓度的对照品溶液。

3. **供试品溶液的制备**　取注射用益气复脉（冻干）样品约 1.0g，精密称定，置 10ml 量瓶中，用 20% 乙腈溶解并稀释至刻度，摇匀，即得。

4. **指纹图谱的建立**

（1）指纹图谱的绘制　分别精密吸取对照品溶液与供试品溶液各 10μl，注入液相色谱仪，测定，记录色谱图。测定各批注射用益气复脉（冻干）样品的指纹图谱，通过"中药色谱指纹图谱相似度评价系统的操作规范（版本2004A）"软件，生成注射液对照指纹图谱，另取10批制剂，与对照指纹图谱进行验证，计算相似度。

（2）共有峰的确定　比较不同批样品的色谱图，确定参比峰，计算各共有指纹峰的相对保留时间及相对峰面积。

（3）共有峰的指认　吸取对照品溶液各10μl，注入液相色谱仪，通过对照品对照法对色谱峰进行指认。

【实验记录】

1. 记录测定数据。

2. 记录实验中出现的问题。

3. 计算共有峰的含量。

【思考题】

1. 用HPLC指纹图谱法对中成药进行质量控制有哪些优点？

2. 如何选择参比峰？

3. 为什么药材麦冬在指纹图谱中没有表现出来？

【相关资料】

1. **注射用益气复脉**　处方：红参提取物、麦冬提取物、五味子提取物。功能与主治：益气生津、敛阴止汗。用于治疗冠心病、劳累性心绞痛、气阴两虚等证。

2. **红参**　来源于五加科植物人参 *Panax ginseng* C. A. Mey. 的干燥根和根茎。主要含有人参皂苷类化合物。

3. **麦冬**　来源于百合科植物麦冬 *Ophiopogon japonicus*（L. f）Ker – Gawl. 的干燥块根。主要含有麦冬皂苷和高异黄酮类化合物和挥发油，但由于甾体皂苷类化合物的含量非常低，高异黄酮类化合物的水溶性差，因此在指纹图谱中不易表现出来。

4. **五味子**　来源于木兰科植物五味子 *Schisandra chinensis*（Turcz.）Baill. 的干燥成熟果实。主要含有五味子素（schizandrin）、去氧五味子素（deoxyschizandrin）、新一味子素（neoschizandrin）、五味子醇（schizan drol）、五味子酯（schisantherin，gomisin）等。

5. **指纹图谱方法学考察**

（1）精密度试验　取同一供试品溶液连续进样5次，分别对各共有峰的相对保留时间及峰面积的变化情况进行考察，计算各共有峰保留时间的RSD值及相对峰面积的RSD值。

（2）重复性试验　取同一批样品制备5份注射剂供试品溶液，分别进样，以13号峰（五味子醇甲）作为参考，考察共有峰的保留时间及相对峰面积，计算各共有峰保留时间的RSD值及相对峰面积的RSD值。

（3）稳定性试验　取同一供试品溶液，分别放置0、4、8、12、24小时进样测定，以13号峰（五味子醇甲）作为参考，考察共有峰的相对保留时间及相对峰面积的变化情况，计算各共有峰保留时间的RSD值及相对峰面积的RSD值。

Experiment 12 HPLC fingerprint chromatography of Yiqifumai Injection

Purpose

1. To master the application of the HPLC fingerprint for the quality control of the Traditional Chinese Medicine (TCM) injection.

2. To be familiar with establishing the HPLC fingerprint method.

Principle

Establish fingerprint chromatography for multiple batches of Yiqifumai Injection by HPLC, using similarity evaluation software evaluated it and determining the reference peak, calculating relative retention time and relative peak area of the common peaks.

Apparatus, Materials and Reagents

1. Apparatus: HPLC, microsyringe.

2. Materials: volumetric flask (10ml), micro - porous filtration member.

3. Reagents: acetontrile (CP), redistilled water, phosphoric acid, methanol (AP).

4. Drugs: ginsenoside Re, Rg_1 CRS, panaxadiol CRS, panaxatriol CRS, schizandrin CRS, deoxyschizandrin CRS, Yiqifumai Injection (for sale).

Experiment contents

1. Chromatographic system and system suitability

Use octadecylsilane bonded silica gel as the stationary phase and a mixture of acetonitrile - 0.05% solution of phosphoric acid as the mobile phase with gradient elution (Shown in table 5 - 1); the wavelength of the detector is 203 nm. The number of theoretical plates of column is not less than 2000, calculated with the reference to the peak of ginsenoside Rg_1.

Table 5 - 1 HPLC gradient elution conditions

Time (min)	A 0.05% phosphoric acid	B acetonitrile
0 - 10	80→70	20→30
10 - 18	70→69	30→31
18 - 30	69→67	31→33
30 - 40	67→55	33→45
40 - 50	55→45	45→55
50 - 70	45→10	55→90

2. Preparation of reference solution

Take some of ginsenoside Re, Rg_1, panaxadiol, panxatriol, schizandrin, deoxy schizandrin, weigh accurately, dissolve in methanol, are prepared by a certain concentration of the reference solution.

3. Preparation of test solution

Take Yiqifumai Injection (lyophilized) about 1. 0 g, weigh accurately, set it into 10 ml volumetric flask, dissolve with 20% acetonitrile and dilute to the mark, shake well, as the test solution.

4. Establishment of the fingerprint

(1) Drawing of the fingerprint Accurately inject 10 μl each of the reference solution and the test solution respectively, into the column and determine, record the chromatograms. Determinate the fingerprint of each batch Yiqifumai Injection (lyophilized), generate injection reference fingerprint through related software, calculate similarity.

(2) Determine of common peaks Compare different batches of samples chromatograms, determine the reference peak and calculate relative retention time and relative peak area of the common peaks.

(3) Identification of common peaks Accurately inject 10 μl each of the reference solution and the test solution respectively, into the column, common peaks are identified by reference control method.

Experiment records

1. Record original data of the experiment.

2. Record the experiment process and the problems.

3. Calculate the content of the common peaks.

Questions

1. HPLC fingerprint method is used for the quality control of the raditional Chinese Medicine (TCM) injection, What are the advantages?

2. How to choose the reference peak?

3. Why Ophiopogonis Radix do not show it in fingerprints ?

Related materials

1. Ingredients of Yiqifumai injection: Ginseng Radix et Rhizoma Rubra extract, Ophiopogonis Radix extract, Schisandrae Chinensis Fructus extract. Action: to supplement qi and promot the production of body fluid, converge yin, and hidroschesis. Indications: coronary heart disease, exertional angina, deficiency of both qi and yin etc.

2. Ginseng Radix et Rhizoma Rubra is the dried root and rhizoma (processed) of *Panax ginseng* C. A. Mey. It's main constituents are ginseng saponin .

3. Ophiopogonis Radix is the dried radix of *Ophiopogon japonicus* (L. f) Ker – Gawl. It's main constituents are ophiopogon saponin, homoisoflavones and volatile oil. But the content of steroidal saponins is very low and homoisoflavones have poor water solubility, therefore they are difficult to show in fingerprints.

4. Schisandrae Chinensis Fructus is the dried mature fruits of *Schisandra chinensis* (Turcz.) Baill. It mainly contains schizandrin, deoxyschizandrin, neoschizandrin, schizandrol, schisantherin etc.

5. Methodology of the study

（1）Precision test Take the same test solution to inject 5 times, respectively, investigate relative retention time and relative peak area of the common peaks, calculate their the value of RSD.

（2）Repeatability test Take 5 sample solution test to inject, respectively. Regard the 13th peak（schizandrol）as a reference, investigate relative retention time and relative peak area of the common peaks, calculate their the value of RSD.

（3）Stability test Take the same test solution, which placed 0, 4, 8, 12, 24h, the sample were determinated as 13th peak（schizandrol）a reference, investigate relative retention time and relative peak area of the common peaks, calculate their the value of RSD.

实验十三 "一测多评"法测定三黄片中4种黄芩黄酮类成分

【目的要求】

1. 掌握"一测多评法"的基本原理。

2. 熟悉高效液相在中药制剂有效成分测定中的应用。

【原理】

一测多评法原理与校正因子法原理基本一致，利用相对保留时间（RT）差和峰形判断目标峰的位置。即在一定的线性范围内成分的量 W（质量或浓度）与检测器响应值 A 成正比（$W = f \cdot A$）。在多指标质量评价时，以样品中某一典型组分（有对照品供应者）为内标，建立该组分与其他组分之间的相对校正因子，通过校正因子计算其他组分的含量。

【仪器、试剂与药品】

1. **仪器** 高效液相色谱仪、超声波清洗器、十万分之一天平、微量进样器。

2. **材料** EP 管、量瓶（50ml）、微孔滤膜、具塞锥形瓶。

3. **试剂** 甲醇（色谱纯）、重蒸水（色谱纯）、磷酸（分析纯）、甲醇（分析纯）。

4. **药品** 黄芩苷对照品、三黄片（市售）。

【实验内容】

1. 色谱条件与系统适用性试验 以十八烷基硅烷键合硅胶为填充剂；甲醇 - 0.2% 磷酸水溶液为流动相（A：甲醇；B：0.2% 磷酸水溶液），梯度洗脱，洗脱程序为：0 ～10min，45% ～ 45% A；10 ～ 55min，45% ～ 70% A，体积流量为 1ml/min，柱温 30℃，检测波长 274nm。理论板数按黄芩苷峰计算应不低于 3000.

2. 对照品溶液的制备 取对照品黄芩苷 10.0mg，精密称定，置 50ml 量瓶中，加甲醇溶解并稀释至刻度，摇匀，配成质量浓度为每 1ml 含黄芩苷 0.20mg 的溶液，即得。

3. 供试品溶液的制备 取本品 10 片，除去包衣，研细，取约 0.1g，精密称定，置具塞锥形瓶中，精密加入 70% 甲醇 25ml，密塞，称定质量，超声处理（功率 250W，工作频率40kHz）10min，取出，放冷，再称定质量，用70%甲醇补足减失的质量，摇匀，用0.22μm微孔滤膜滤过，取续滤液，即得。

4. 测定法 分别精密吸取对照品溶液与供试品溶液各10μl，注入液相色谱仪，测定，即得。本品每片含黄芩浸膏以黄芩苷（$C_{12}H_{18}O_{11}$）计，小片不得少于13.5mg，大片不得少于27mg。

【实验记录】

1. 记录测定数据。

2. 记录实验中出现的问题。

3. 计算三黄片中4种黄酮类成分的含量。

【思考题】

1. 用一测多评法测定中成药有效成分的主要优势是什么？

2. 用超声提取法提取黄芩苷有哪些优点？

3. 为什么取续滤液作为供试品溶液？否则对结果有何影响？

【相关资料】

1. **三黄片** 处方：大黄300g，盐酸小檗碱5g，黄芩浸膏21g（相当于黄芩苷15g）。制法：黄芩浸膏系取黄芩，加水煎煮三次，第一次1.5小时，第二次1小时，第三次40分钟，合并煎液，滤过，滤液加盐酸调节pH至1~2，静置1小时，取沉淀，用水洗涤使pH至5~7，烘干，粉碎成细粉，测定含量，备用。取大黄150g，粉碎成细粉，过筛；剩余大黄粉碎成粗粉，加30%乙醇回流提取3次，滤过，合并滤液，回收乙醇并减压浓缩至稠膏状，加入大黄细粉、盐酸小檗碱细粉、黄芩浸膏细粉及辅料适量，混匀，制成颗粒，干燥，压制成1000片，包糖衣，即得。功能与主治：清热解毒，泻火通便，用于三焦热盛所致的目赤肿痛、口鼻生疮、咽喉肿痛、牙龈肿痛、心烦口渴、尿黄、便秘；亦用于急性胃肠炎，痢疾。

2. **黄芩** 为唇形科植物黄芩（*Scutellaria baicalensis* Georgi），以根入药。主含黄酮类成分，如黄芩苷、汉黄芩苷、黄芩素、汉黄芩素。

其中结构如下：

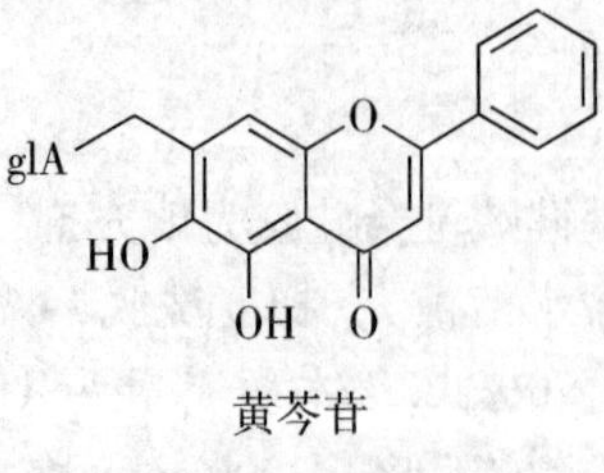

黄芩苷 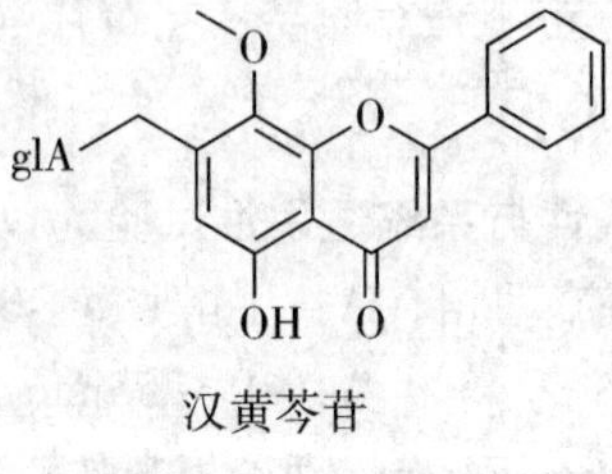　　　　　　　　　　　汉黄芩苷

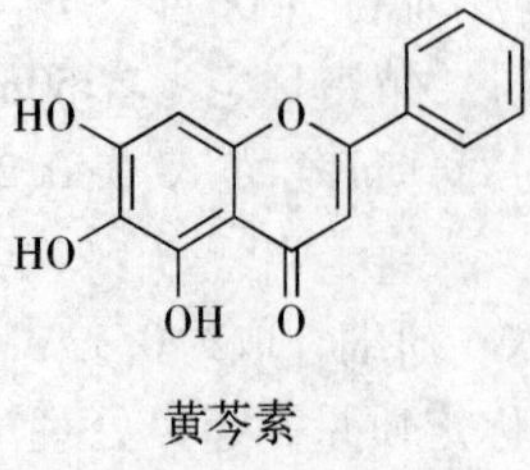

黄芩素 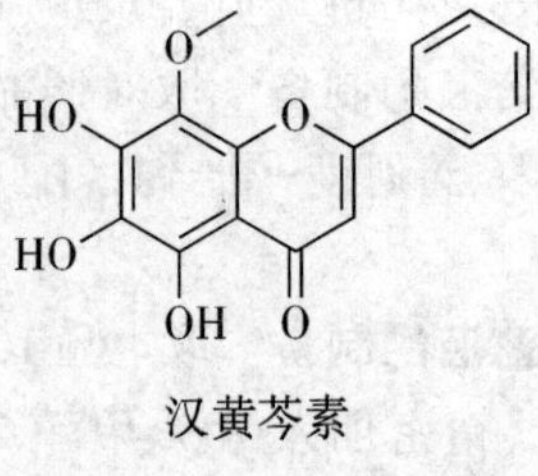　　　　　　　　　　　汉黄芩素

3. 黄芩黄酮类成分间相对校正因子 分别为 $f_A^{274nm} = 1.20$，$f_B^{274nm} = 1.62$，$f_C^{274nm} = 1.68$，其中：A 为汉黄芩苷/黄芩苷、B 为黄芩素/黄芩苷、C 为汉黄芩素/黄芩苷。见图 5 – 5。

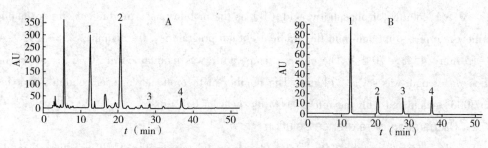

图 5 – 5 三黄片供试品 HPLC 图（A）和对照品 HPLC 图（B）
1. 黄芩苷 2. 汉黄芩苷 3. 黄芩素 4. 汉黄芩素

Experiment 13 Determination of four kinds of Scutellaria flavonoids in Sanhuang Tablets by QAMS

Purpose

1. To master the basic principles of QAMS.

2. To master the application of HPLC in assay of effective ingredients of Chinese medicine preparation.

Principle

The principles of Quantitative Assay of Multi – components by Single – marker（QAMS）and the relative correction factor method are almost the same, using the relative retention time（RT）and peak shape to judge the position of the target peak. That is, in a certain amount of the component within the linear range W（weight or concentration）is proportional to the detector response values A（$W = f \cdot A$）. In the multi – maker quality assessment to a typical constituents of the sample（with reference Publishers）as the internal standard, the establishment of the relative correction factor of the component and the other components, then calculated the content of other components by correction factor.

Apparatus, materials, reagents and drugs

1. Appatatus：HPLC, ultrasonic surge, microsyringe, Hundred thousandth analytical balance；

2. Materials：EP tube, volumetric flask（50 ml）, micro porous filtration member stoppered conical flask.

3. Reagents：methanol（CP）, redistilled water（CP）, phosphoric acid（AP）, methanol（AP）.

4. Drugs：baicalin CRS；Sanhuang Tablets（for sale）.

Experiment contents

1. Chromatographic system and system suitability

Use octadecylsilane bonded silica gel as the stationary phase and a mixture of methaol (A) −0. 2% solution of phosphoric acid (B) as the mobile phase in gradient elution manner at a flow rate of 1. 0 ml/min and the gradient elution program is: 0 − 10 min, 45% − 45% A; 10 − 55 min, 45% − 70% A. The column temperature was maintained at 30 ℃, and the detection wavelength was set at 274 nm. The number of theoretical plates of column is not less than 3000, calculated with the reference to the peak of baicalin.

2. Preparation of reference solution

Dissolve some of baicalin CRS, weighed accurately, with methanol. The solution contains 0. 20 mg of baicalin per ml.

3. Preparation of test solution

Take this product 10 to remove the coating, porphyrized, then take about 0. 1 g, accurately weighed, and set stoppered Erlenmeyer flask, add 25 ml of 70% methanol in a stopped concial flask, stopper tightly and weigh. Ultrasonicate for 10 minutes (power, 250 W; frequency, 40 kHz), cool to ambient temperature and weigh again. Replenish the lost weight with 70% ethanol, mix well, filter and use the successive filtrate.

4. Assay

Accurately inject 10 μl each of the reference solution and the test solution, respectively, into the column and determine. It contains not less than 13. 5 mg of baicalin ($C_{12}H_{18}O_{11}$) for each small piece and 27. 0 mg for large tracts.

Experiment records

1. Make record of the experiment.

2. Record the difficulties encountered.

3. Calculate the contents of four kinds of Scutellaria flavonoids.

Questions

1. What is the main advantage of determination of Chinese medicine preparation effective components by QAMS ?

2. What are the advantages of Ultrasonic extraction method to extract baicalin?

3. Why do we take the successive filtrate as the test solution?

Related materials

1. Ingredients of Sanhuang Tablets: Rhei Radix et Rhizoma 300 g, Berberine Hydrochloride 5 g, Scutellariae Extract 21 g (containing about 15 g of baicalin). Method: the preparation of Scutellariae Extract——take Scutellariae Radix, add boiling water three times, the first 1. 5 hours, the second one hour, the third 40 minutes, combined decoction, filtration, The filtrate was added hydrochloric acid to adjust the pH value to 1 − 2, for 1 hours, the precipitate was washed with water to make the pH value to 5 − 7, drying, pulverizing into fine powder, the

content was determined, spare. Rhei Radix et Rhizoma 150 g, crushed into fine powder, sifted; Rhei Radix et Rhizoma remaining crushed into coarse powder, plus 30% ethanol extraction three times, filtration, combined filtrate recovery of ethanol and concentrated under reduced pressure to a thick paste, adding Rhei Radix et Rhizoma powder, hydrochloric acid berberine powder, Extraction of Scutellariae Radix powder and excipients amount, mixing, granulating, drying, pressing into 1000, including sugar, that was. Actions: To clear heat, remove toxin, purge fire and open the bowels. Indications: Pattern of exuberant heat in the triple, manifested as red painful swelling eyes, mouth and nose sores, sores throat and gums, vexation, thirst, yellow – colored urine and constipation; Acute gastroenteritis or dysentery with the symptoms described above.

2. Scutellariae Radixis the dried root of *Scutellaria baicalensis* Georgi. It's main constituents are flavonoids, such as baicalin, wogonoside, baicalein, wogonin. And the chemical structure are as follow:

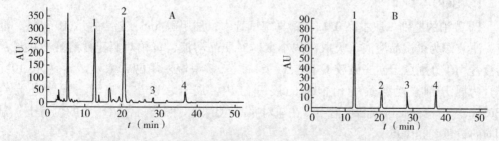

3. The relative correction factor of Scutellaria flavonoids is $f_A^{274nm} = 1.20$ $f_B^{274nm} = 1.62$ $f_C^{274nm} = 1.68$, Where in: A is wogonoside / baicalin, B is baicalein / baicalin, C is Wogonin / baicalin. (Figure 5 – 5)

Figure 5 – 5 HPLC chromatogram of Sanhuang Tablets (A) and HPLC chromatogram of the reference (B)

1. Baicalin 2. wogonoside 3. Baicalein 4. Wogonin

第六章 综合性实验

Chapter 6　Comprehensive Experiment

实验十四　二妙丸的鉴别与挥发油的测定

【目的要求】

1. 掌握薄层色谱法在中成药鉴别中的应用。

2. 熟悉挥发油测定方法。

【原理】

采用薄层色谱法，以对照品和对照药材作对照，鉴别中成药的处方。利用挥发油可随水蒸气蒸馏的性质测定挥发油的含量。《中国药典》中挥发油的测定有两种方法，甲法适用于测定相对密度在1.0以下的挥发油，乙法适用于测定相对密度在1.0以上的挥发油。采用薄层色谱法分析挥发油的组成。

【仪器、试剂与药品】

1. **仪器**　挥发油测定器、紫外灯（365nm）、超声波清洗器。

2. **材料**　冷凝管（24#）、圆底烧瓶（24#）、硅胶G薄层板（5cm×10cm）2块、立式展开槽（10cm×10cm）、滤纸、小漏斗、具塞试管（10ml）、试管、毛细管、玻璃珠、烧杯、干燥小瓶、钢铲。

3. **试剂**　乙醚、石油醚（60～90℃）、乙酸乙酯、三氯甲烷、甲醇、浓氨试液、5%香草醛硫酸溶液、无水硫酸钠。

4. **药品**　盐酸小檗碱对照品溶液（0.5mg/ml）；黄柏对照药材溶液（0.1g加甲醇5ml超声10分钟）；二妙丸（市售品）。

【实验内容】

1. **黄柏的鉴别**　取本品0.1g，置具塞试管中，加甲醇5ml，超声提取10分钟，滤过，滤液作为供试品溶液。吸取盐酸小檗碱对照品溶液、黄柏对照药材溶液及供试品溶液各5μl分别点于同一硅胶G薄层板上，以三氯甲烷-甲醇-浓氨试液（50:10:0.5）为展开剂，置氨蒸气预饱和的展开缸内，展开，取出，晾干，置紫外光灯（365nm）下检视。供试品色谱中，在与对照品色谱及对照药材色谱相应的位置上，显相同的黄色荧光斑点。

2. **挥发油的测定**　取烧瓶，加水300ml与玻璃珠数粒，称取供试品约60g，置烧瓶中，振摇混合后，连接挥发油测定器与冷凝管。从冷凝管上端加水约200ml，使充满挥发油测定器的刻度部分，并溢流入烧瓶为止。用直火缓缓加热至沸，并保持微沸1小时，停止加热，放置片刻，开启测定器下端的活塞，将水缓缓放出，至油层下降至其上端恰与刻度 0 线平齐，读取挥发油量，并计算供试品中挥发油的含量（%）。

$$挥发油含量 = V / W \times 100\%$$

式中，V——挥发油的体积（ml）；

W——供试品的重量（g）。

3. 苍术挥发油组成　吸取挥发油少量，置干燥小瓶中，加乙醚 1ml，加少量无水硫酸钠，上清液作为供试品溶液。吸取供试品溶液 5μl，点于硅胶 G 薄层板上，以石油醚（60~90℃）－乙酸乙酯（85：15）为展开剂，展开，取出，晾干，喷以 5% 香草醛硫酸溶液，供试品的色谱中，出现橙红色、污绿色两个主斑点。

【实验记录】

1. 绘制黄柏鉴别的薄层色谱图。

2. 绘制挥发油测定仪器，记录实验中的重要步骤及出现的问题，计算本品挥发油的含量。

3. 绘制苍术挥发油薄层色谱图。

【思考题】

1. 本法测定挥发油的原理是什么？若挥发油相对密度为 1.0 以上如何设计实验？

2. 挥发油测定的意义是什么？

3. 什么是对照品和对照药材？

【相关资料】

1. **二妙丸**　处方：苍术（炒）500g 与黄柏（炒）500g。制法：粉碎，过筛，混匀，水泛丸，干燥，即得。功能与主治：燥湿清热，用于湿热下注，足膝红肿热痛，下肢丹毒，白带，阴囊湿痒。

2. **苍术**　为菊科植物茅苍术 *Atractylodes lancea* Thunb. DC. 或北苍术 *Atractylodes chinensis* DC. Koidz. 的干燥根茎。苍术挥发油中主要含有苍术酮（atractylon）、苍术素（atractylodin）、β－桉油醇（eudesmol）、茅术醇（hinesol）等。经香草醛浓硫酸显色后，苍术酮显橙红色，苍术素显污绿色，β－桉油醇和茅术醇显紫红色。

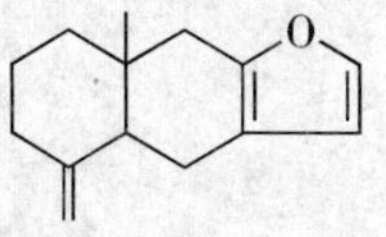

苍术酮

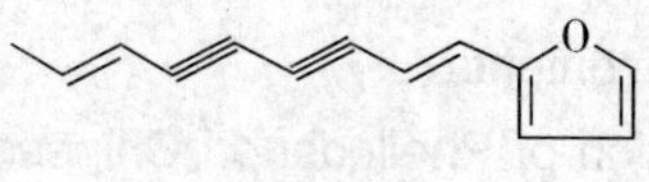

苍术素

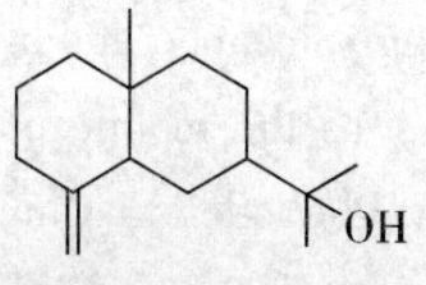

β－桉油醇

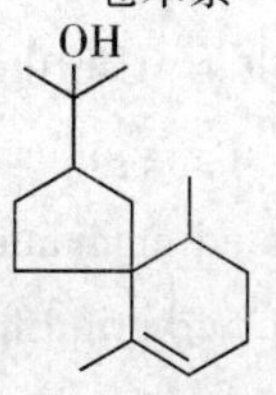

茅术醇

黄柏为芸香科植物黄皮树 *Phellodendron Chinens* Schneid. 的干燥树皮。主要含有小檗碱、药根碱、巴马亭碱、黄连碱等生物碱。

Experiment 14   Identification of Ermiao Pills and

Determination of Volatile Oil

Purpose

1. To master the common analysis method applied in identification and determination of Traditional Chinese patent medicines.

2. To be familiar with the method for V. O. determination.

Principle

Chemical reference substance and reference drug are used in TLC method to identify CT-PM (Traditional Chinese patent medicine). The V. O. can be extracted and determined by vapour distillation method due to its characteristic of vapouring with steam. There are two methods for determining the V. O. in Chinese pharmacopeia. Method one is applied to determine the V. O. whom density is less than 1.0 and method two is applied to determine the V. O. of whom density is more than 1.0.

TLC method is used to analyze the ingredients of the V. O.

Apparatus, materials, reagents and drugs

1. Apparatus: V. O. determination tube, ultraviolet lamp (365 nm), ultrasonic surge.

2. Materials: condenser tube ($24^\#$), round flask ($24^\#$), two pieces of silica gel G plate (5 cm × 10 cm), vertical developing chamber (10 cm × 10 cm), filter paper, small hopper, stoppered tube (10 ml), tube, capillary, beading, beaker, dried bottle, steel shovel.

3. Reagents: ethyl ether, petroleum ether (60 – 90 ℃), ethyl acetate, chloroform, methanol, concentrated ammonia TS, 5% vanillin sulfate solution, anhydrous sodium sulfate.

4. Drugs: berberine hydrochloride CRS (0.5 mg/ml); reference substance of Phellodendri Chinensis Cortex CRS (0.1 g add 5 ml of methanol, ultrasonicate 10 minutes); Ermiao Pills (for sale).

Experiment contents

1. Identification of Phellodendri Chinensis Cortex

To 0.1 g of the sample, place in a stoppered test tube, add 5 ml of methanol, ultrasonicate for 10 minutes, and filter. Use the filtrate as the test solution. Carry out the method for thin layer chromatography, using silica gel G as the coating substance and a mixture of chloroform – methanol – concentrated ammonia TS (50: 10: 0.5) as the mobile phase. Apply separately to plate 5 μl each of berberine hydrochloride CRS, Phellodendri Chinensis Cortex CRS solution and the test solution. After developing in a chamber pre – equilibrated with ammonia vapour for 15 minutes, and removal of the plate, dry it in air, examine under ultraviolet light (365 nm). The yellow fluorescent spots in the chromatogram obtained with the test solution corresponds to that obtained with the reference solution and the reference drug solution.

2. The determination of the V. O.

Fill the flask with 300 ml of water and several beadings, weigh 60 g of test sample, place it in the flask, after shaking and mixing, connect the V. O. detector and condenser tube. Add about 200 ml of water from the top of the condenser tube, don't stop until the water full of the scale of the V. O. extractor. Heat mildly till the water boiling, and maintain for 1 hour, then stop and unfold the piston at the bottom of the detector later, let the water flow out slowly until the oil layer descending to the zero, read the volume of V. O. and calculate the content of V. O. of the test.

$$\text{Content of V. O.} = V/W \times 100\%$$

V——the volume of V. O. (ml);

W——the weigh of test (g).

3. The ingredients of the V. O. in Atractylodis Rhizoma

Place a little V. O. in a dry bottle, add 1 ml of ethyl ether and a little anhydrous sodium sulfate, use supernatant as the test solution. Take 5 μl of test solution, and apply to plate coated with silica gel G, using the mixture of petroleum ether (60 – 90 ℃) – ethyl acetate (85:15) as developing solution, develop, removal, dry, spray 5% vanillin sulfate solution, then there are two chief spots on the test solution plate with the colour of orange and dark green.

Experiment records

1. Draw the TLC chromatogram of indentification of Phellodendri Chinensis Cortex.

2. Draw apparatus of determinating volatile oil. Record the necessary procedure of the experiment and the problem.

3. Draw the TLC chromatogram of V. O. inrhizome astractylodis.

Questions

1. What's the principle of determination of V. O. ? How to design a determination experiment for V. O. which density is more than 1.0?

2. What is the meaning of determination result of the V. O. ?

3. What's the meaning of CRS and reference drug?

Related materials

1. Ingredients of Ermiao Pills: Atractylodis Rhizoma (stir – baked) 500 g and Phellodendri Chinensis Cortex (stir – baked) 500 g. Procedure: pulverize the two ingredients to fine powder, sift and mix well. Make pills with water and dry. Action: To remove damp – heat. Indication: damp – heat in the lower part of the body marked by redness, swelling, hotness and pain in the legs and knees, erysipelas of the lower extremities, morbid leucorrhea, or wetness and itching of the scrotum.

2. Atractylodis comes from the dried rhizoma of *Atractylodes lancea* Thunb. DC. or *Atractylodes chinensis* DC. Koidz. Its component of V. O. is complex e. g. atractylon, atractylodin, eudesmol, hinesol. After coloration by vanillin – concentrated sulfate solution, it appears different colors. There are three chief spots, one is generated by atractylon (orange), the other is generated by atractylodin (dark green), and the third is generated by eudesmol and hinesol (fuchsia).

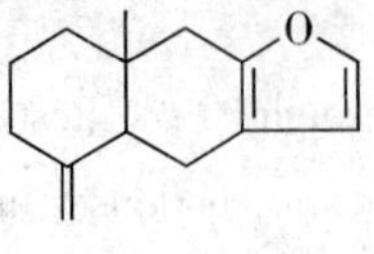

atractylon

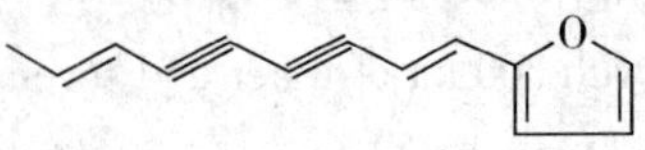

atractylodin

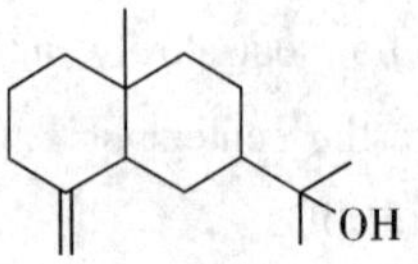

eudesmol

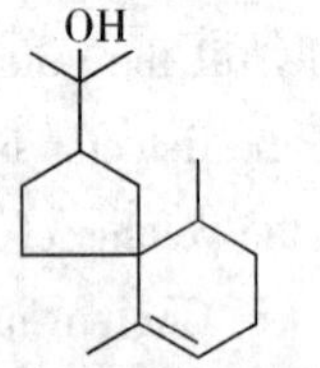

hinesol

Phellodendron is from the dried cortex of *Phellodendron Chinens* Schneid（Rutaceae）. It mainly contains alkaloids such as berbeine，jateorrhizine，palmatine and coptisine.

实验十五 大山楂丸的鉴别与总黄酮的含量测定

【目的要求】

1. 掌握常用分析方法在中成药鉴别与含量测定中的应用。
2. 熟悉总黄酮类成分含量测定的原理和方法。

【原理】

大山楂丸中山楂主要含有机酸和黄酮类成分，可以此作为定性定量依据；而麦芽和神曲的显微特征明显，可以作为鉴别依据。

山楂中黄酮类成分的结构具有 C_3-OH、C_5-OH 或 $3',4'$ 邻二酚羟基的黄酮类，能与金属离子 Al^{3+}、Mg^{2+}、Zr^{2+} 等产生较稳定的颜色反应，吸收一定波长的可见光。本实验以与山楂中总黄酮结构类似的槲皮素（也具有 C_3-OH、C_5-OH）为对照品，从槲皮素标准曲线读出总黄酮的量，换算出成药中总黄酮的含量。

【仪器、试剂与药品】

1. **仪器** 分光光度计、超声波清洗器、显微镜。
2. **材料** 硅胶 G 薄层板（5cm×10cm）、立式展开槽（10cm×10cm）、量瓶（50ml、10ml）、锥形瓶（50ml）、刻度移液管（5ml、2ml、1ml）、滴管、试管、烧杯、载玻片、盖玻片、酒精灯、乳钵、滤纸、棉花、擦镜纸、小镊子、小刀。
3. **试剂** 蒸馏水、乙醇（50%、95%）、盐酸、乙酸乙酯、正丁醇、甲醇、三氯甲烷、丙酮、5%亚硝酸钠溶液、1mol/L 氢氧化钠溶液、10%硝酸铝溶液、10%硫酸乙醇溶液、水合氯醛试液、稀甘油、镁粉。
4. **药品** 槲皮素对照品溶液（0.2mg/ml），熊果酸对照品溶液（1.0mg/ml）（中国食品药品检定研究院）；大山楂丸（市售品）。

【实验内容】

1. 鉴别

（1）取本品 1 丸，切碎，120℃干燥 2 小时，放冷至室温，粉碎至细粉，取少许细粉用水合氯醛试液透化后滴加适量稀甘油，置显微镜下观察。

（2）取本品 4.5g，剪碎，加乙醇 20ml，加热 10 分钟，滤过。取滤液 1ml，加少量镁粉与浓盐酸 2～3 滴，加热 4～5 分钟后，即显橙红色。

（3）取（2）项下溶液蒸干，残渣加水 5ml，加热使溶解，加乙酸乙酯 5ml 振摇提取 2 次，合并乙酸乙酯液，蒸干，残渣加甲醇 2ml 使溶解，作为供试品溶液。另取熊果酸对照品，加甲醇制成每 1ml 含 1mg 的溶液，作为对照品溶液。吸取上述两种溶液各 2 μl，分别点于同一硅胶 G 薄层板上，以三氯甲烷－丙酮（9∶1）为展开剂，展开，取出，晾干，喷以 10% 硫酸乙醇溶液，在 105℃ 加热数分钟。供试品色谱中，在与对照品色谱相应的位置上，显相同的紫红色斑点。

2. 含量测定

（1）标准曲线的绘制　精密量取 0.2mg/ml 的槲皮素对照品溶液 0.0、1.0、2.0、3.0、4.0、5.0ml，分别置于 10ml 量瓶中，各加 50% 乙醇溶液至 5ml，精密加 5% 亚硝酸钠溶液 0.3ml，摇匀，放置 6 分钟，加入 10% 硝酸铝溶液 0.3ml，再放置 6 分钟，加入 1mol/L 氢氧化钠溶液 4ml，再加 50% 乙醇溶液至刻度，摇匀，放置 15 分钟，以相应试剂为空白，置比色杯中，于 500nm 波长处测定吸光度，以吸光度为纵坐标，浓度为横坐标，绘制标准曲线。

（2）供试品溶液的制备　取 120℃ 干燥 2 小时的大山楂丸粗粉 1.0g，置 50ml 锥形瓶中，加 95% 乙醇 20ml，超声提取 15 分钟，滤过；滤渣再加 50% 乙醇 10ml，超声提取 5 分钟，滤过，合并滤液，移入 50ml 量瓶中，放凉至室温，补加蒸馏水至刻度，摇匀，即得。

（3）测定法　精密吸取供试品溶液 1ml，置 10ml 量瓶中，以下同标准曲线项下操作，测定其吸光度，由标准曲线中读出供试品中槲皮素的含量，即得，计算大山楂丸中总黄酮的含量。

【实验记录】

1. 绘出显微鉴别图。

2. 绘出薄层色谱图。

3. 绘制标准曲线。

4. 计算总黄酮的含量。

【思考题】

1. 采用本方法所测定的总黄酮含量是相对含量还是绝对含量？说明结果的意义。

2. 影响本实验含量测定准确性的因素有哪些？

【相关资料】

1. 大山楂丸　处方：山楂 1000g，六神曲（焦）150g，麦芽（炒）150g。制法：以上三味，粉碎，过筛，混匀。取蔗糖 600g，加水 270ml 与炼蜜 600g，混合，滤过，煎煮至相对密度为 1.38（70℃），与上述粉末混匀，制成大蜜丸，即得。功能与主治：开胃消食。用于食积内停所致的食欲不振、消化不良、脘腹胀闷。

2. 山楂　来源于蔷薇科植物山里红 *Crataegus pinnatifida* Bge. var. *major* N. E. Br. 或山楂 *Crataegus pinnatifida* Bge. 的干燥成熟果实，主要成分为有机酸、黄酮类及多种维生素。黄酮类化合物主要为金丝桃苷、牡荆素等，有机酸主要有乌苏酸、齐墩果酸、山楂酸等。

金丝桃苷

乌苏酸

牡荆素

3. 六神曲 六神曲中的小麦的粉末特征为：淀粉粒单粒类圆形，略扁，直径约至 43μm，脐点呈长裂缝状；复粒较小，由 2~6 分粒组成。横细胞表面观呈长条形，直径 7~22μm，长 40~243μm，垂周壁连珠状增厚。

4. 麦芽 粉末特征为：秤片外表皮淡黄色，表面观由长细胞与两个短细胞相间排列。长细胞长条形，壁厚，深波状弯曲。如图 6-1 所示。

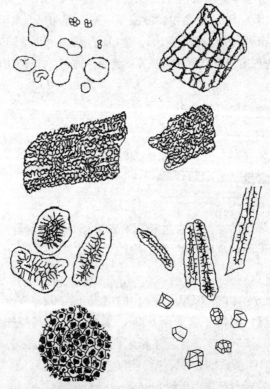

图 6-1 大山楂丸显微鉴别图

1. 六神曲（小麦：a. 淀粉粒；b. 果皮横细胞及管细胞） 2. 麦芽（秤片外表皮表面观）

3. 山楂（a. 石细胞；b. 纤维；c. 果皮表皮细胞；d. 方晶）

5. 试剂的配制

（1）水合氯醛试液　取水合氯醛 50g，加水 15ml 与甘油 10ml 使溶解，即得。

（2）稀甘油　取甘油 33ml，加水稀释使成 100ml，再加樟脑一小块或液化苯酚 1 滴，即得。

Experiment 15　Identification of Dashanzha Pills and Determination of Total Flavonoids

Purpose

1. To master the method of frequently – used analytic method in the identification and assay of Traditional Chinese patent medicines and the assay.

2. To be familiar with the principle and the method of the determination of the total flavonoids.

Principle

There are organic acid and flavonoids in Chinese hawthorn which can be used as basis of quality and quantities identification. Evident microscopical characters in malt and medicated leaven can be used to identify.

Flavonoids in Chinese hawthorn have $C_3 - OH$、$C_5 - OH$ or $3', 4' -$ dihydroxy, and rutin has similar groups and could be used as reference substance which can react with Al^{3+}、Mg^{2+}、Zr^{2+} and so on, produce stable color reaction, and absorb the visible light. The reaction has high sensitivity and good selectivity. From the standard curve of rutin we can calculate the concentration of the total flavonoids.

Apparatus, materials, reagents and drugs

1. Apparatus: spectrophotometer, ultrasonic surge, microscope.

2. Materials: silica gel G – TLC plate (5 cm × 10 cm), vertical developing chamber (10 cm × 10 cm), volumetric flask (50 ml, 10 ml), conical flack (50 ml), measuring pipette (5 ml, 2 ml, 1 ml), dropper, test – tube, beaker, microscope slide, cave glass, alcohol burner, forceps, filter paper, absorbent cotton, knife.

3. Reagents: distilled water, alcohol (50%, 95%), n – butanol, methanol, chloroform, acetone, 5% sodium nitrite, sodium hydrate (1 mol/L), 10% aluminium nitrate, 10% sulfuric acid in alcohol, chloral hydrate TS, glycerin dilute TS, magnesium powder, hydrochloric acid, acetate.

4. Drugs: solution of quercetin CRS (0. 2 mg/ml), solution of ursolic acid CRS (1. 0 mg/ml); Dashanzha Pills (for sale).

Experiment contents

1. Identification

（1）To 1 pill, cut into pieces, dry for 2 hours at 120 ℃, cool to ambient temperature, grind to fine powder. To some fine powder, add chloral hydrate TS to heat. Afterward, drop some dilute glycerin and observe under the microscope.

(2) To 4.5 g of pills, cut into pieces, add 20 ml of ethanol, heat for 10 minutes, filter. To 1 ml of the filtrate add a small quantity of magnesium powder and 2 – 3 drops of hydrochloric acid, heat for 4 – 5 minutes, and orange – red color is produced.

(3) Place the liquid in (2) to dryness, dissolve the residue in 5 ml of water on heating, extract twice with 5 ml of ethyl acetate, shaking. Combine the ethyl acetate solution and evaporate to dryness, dissolve the residue in 2 ml of methanol as the test solution. Dissolve ursolic acid CRS in methanol to produce a solution containing 1 mg per ml as the reference solution. Using silica gel G as the coating substance and a mixture of chloroform – acetone (9 : 1) as the mobile phase. Apply separately to the plate 2 μl each of the above two solutions. After developing and removal of the plate, dry it in air. Spray with a 10% solution of sulfuric acid in ethanol and heat at 105 ℃ for several minutes. The purplish – red spot in the chromatogram obtained with the test solution corresponds in position and colour to the spot in the chromatogram obtained with the reference solution.

2. Assay

(1) Preparation of standard curve   Measure accurately 0.0, 1.0, 2.0, 3.0, 4.0 and 5.0 ml of the rutin reference solution, to 10 ml volumetric flasks, add 50% alcohol solution to 5 ml, accurately add 0.3 ml of 50% sodium nitrite solution, mix well. Allow to stand for 6 minutes, add 0.3 ml of 10% aluminium nitrate solution, and allow to stand for 6 minutes, add 4 ml of 1 mol/L sodium hydrate solution, dilute with 50% alcohol solution to volume, mix well. Allow to stand for 15 minutes, pull them into cell. Measure the absorbance of the solution at 500 nm, using solvent as the blank, plot the concentration to absorbance standard curve.

(2) Preparation of test solution   Weigh 1.0 g of Dashanzha Pill, previously dried at 120℃ for 2 hours, to a 50 ml volumetric flask and add 20 ml of 95% alcohol solution, ultrasonic for 15 minutes, filter, dissolve the residue in 10 ml of 50% alcohol, ultrasonic extract for 5 minutes, filter, merged filtrate, transfer the obtained into 50 ml volumetric flask, cool it to room temperature, dilute with water to volume, mix well for use.

(3) Procedure   Measuring accurately 1.0 ml of test solution, to 10 ml volumetric flask. Proceed as described under preparation of standard curve, measuring the absorbance. Calculate content of total flavonoids in Dashanzha Pills with standard curve of quercetin.

Experiment records

1. Draw the micrograph of Dashanzha Pills.

2. Draw the TLC Chromatogram.

3. Draw the standard curve.

4. Calculate the content of total flavonoids inDashanzha Pills.

Questions

1. The content of the total flavonoids determined with the method is relative content or not?

2. Which factors will affect the accuracy of content determination in this experiment?

Related materials

1. Ingredients of Dashanzha Pill: Crataegi Fructus 1000 g, Massa Medicata Fermentata (stir – baked with bran) 150 g, Hordei Fructus Germinatus (stir – baked) 150 g. Procedure: pulverize the above three ingredients to fine powder, sift and mix well. To 600 g of sucrose add 270 ml of water and 600 g of refined honey, mix well. Decoct gently to a relative density of 1.38 (70 ℃), filter, mix well with the above powder to make big honey pills. Action: To boost appetite and promote digestion. Indications: Poor appetite, indigestion, distension and fullness in the epigastrium and abdomen due to internal food retention.

2. Crataegi Fructus is the dried ripe fruit of *Crataegus pinnatifida* Bge. var. *major* N. E. Br. or *Crataegus Pinnatifida* Bge. Its main content are organic acid, flavonoids and varial vitamine. The mainly flavonoids are hyperoside and vitexin, and the mainly organic acid are ursolic acid, oleanolic acid and crataegolic acid.

hyperoside

ursolic acid

vitexin

3. The character of the powder of wheat inmedicated leaven: starch granules simple, subrounded, somewhat flat, about 43 μm in diameter, hilum long cleft; compound granules less, of 2 – 6 components. Cross cell elongated in surface view, 7 – 22μm in diameter, 40 – 243 μm in length, with boaded anticlinal walls.

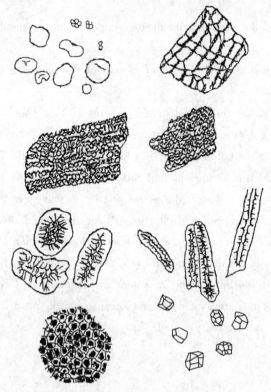

Figure 6 – 1   Microscopical Identification of Dashanzha Pills

1. Massa Medicate Fermentata (wheat：a. starch ranules；b. cross cell and solenocyte of seedcase)

2. Hordei Fructus Germinatus (outface of malt in surface view)   3. Crataegi Fructus (a. stone cells；b. faber；c. carp epidermis cells；d. solitary crystals)   4. The character of the powder

rdei Fructus Germinatus：the outface of the lemma is pale yellow, there are long cells and short cells in surface view. Long cells elongated, wall thickened, deep sinuous. (Figure 6 – 1)

5. Preparation of test solution

(1) Chloral hydrate TS   Dissolve 50 g of chloral hydrate in a mixture of 15 ml of water and 10 ml of glycerin.

(2) Glycerine dilute TS   Dilute 33 ml of glycerine with water to 100 ml. Add a small piece of camphor or a drop of liquefied phenol.

实验十六 双黄连口服液的质量分析

【目的要求】

1. 掌握 HPLC 法测定中药复方中有效成分的方法。

2. 掌握注射剂杂质检查的目的、原理及操作方法。

【原理】

利用薄层色谱法，以对照品和对照药材作对照鉴别中成药的处方。杂质检查项目主要包括：蛋白质检查（加磺基水杨酸或鞣酸检查）、鞣质检查（加鸡蛋清或明胶氯化钠试液检查）、重金属检查（照《中国药典》方法检查，不得超过百万分之十）、砷盐检查（照《中国药典》方法检查，不得超过百万分之二）、草酸盐检查（加氯化钙检查）、钾离子检查（加四苯硼酸钠检查）、树脂检查（加盐酸或冰醋酸检查）。利用HPLC法测定绿原酸和黄芩苷的含量，分别以绿原酸和黄芩苷的最大紫外吸收波长作为检测波长。

【仪器、试剂与药品】

1. 仪器 高效液相色谱仪、超声波清洗器、紫外灯、马弗炉。

2. 材料 硅胶G薄层板（5cm×10cm）、聚酰胺薄膜（5cm×7.5cm）、立式展开槽（10cm×10cm）、漏斗、分液漏斗、量瓶（25ml）、纳氏比色管、毛细管、试管、滤纸。

3. 试剂 甲醇（色谱纯）、75%甲醇、冰醋酸、三氯甲烷、蒸馏水、10%硫酸乙醇溶液、鞣酸试液、稀醋酸、氯化钠明胶试液、盐酸、稀氢氧化钠、3%氯化钙溶液、酚酞指示液、醋酸盐缓冲液（pH 3.5）、标准钾离子溶液、标准砷溶液、标准铅溶液、碱性甲醛溶液、3%乙二胺四醋酸二钠溶液、3%四苯硼钠溶液、三乙胺。

4. 药品 黄芩苷对照品的75%甲醇溶液（0.1mg/ml）、黄芩苷对照品的50%甲醇溶液（0.05mg/ml）、绿原酸对照品的75%甲醇溶液（0.1mg/ml）、绿原酸对照品水溶液（0.02mg/ml）、连翘对照药材溶液（取0.5g，加甲醇5ml，超声处理20分钟）；注射用双黄连（冻干）（市售品）。

【实验内容】

1. 鉴别

（1）黄芩与金银花的鉴别 取本品60mg，加75%甲醇3ml，超声处理使溶解，作为供试品溶液。另分别取黄芩0.1g、连翘0.2g，加75%甲醇5ml，超声提取10分钟，作为金银花阴性对照液；分别取金银花0.1g、连翘0.2g，加75%甲醇5ml，超声提取10分钟，作为黄芩阴性对照液；吸取黄芩苷对照品的75%甲醇溶液、绿原酸对照品的75%甲醇溶液及上述三种溶液各1μl，分别点于同一聚酰胺薄膜上，以醋酸为展开剂，展开，取出，晾干，置紫外光灯（365nm）下检视。供试品色谱中，在与对照品色谱相应的位置上，显相同颜色的荧光斑点。

（2）连翘的鉴别 取本品0.1g，加甲醇5ml，超声处理20分钟，放置，取上清液作为供试品溶液。吸取连翘对照药材溶液及供试品溶液各10μl，分别点于同一以羧甲基纤维素钠为黏合剂的硅胶G板上，以三氯甲烷-甲醇（20:1）为展开剂，展开，取出，晾干，喷以10%硫酸乙醇溶液，在100℃加热至斑点显色清晰。供试品色谱中，在与对照药材色谱相应的位置上，显相同颜色的斑点。

2. 检查

（1）蛋白质 取本品0.1g，置试管中，加水2ml超声使溶解，滴加鞣酸试液1~3滴，不得产生浑浊。

（2）鞣质 取本品0.1g，置试管中，加水2ml超声使溶解，加稀醋酸1滴，再加氯化钠明胶试液4~5滴，不得出现浑浊或沉淀。

(3) 树脂 取本品 0.3g，置试管中，加水 5ml 使溶解，置分液漏斗中，加三氯甲烷 10ml 振摇提取，分取三氯甲烷液，置水浴上蒸干，残渣加冰醋酸 2ml 使溶解，置具塞试管中，加水 3ml，混匀，放置 30 分钟，应无絮状物析出。

(4) 草酸盐 取本品 0.1g，置试管中，加水 2ml 超声使溶解，用稀盐酸调 pH 1 ~ 2，滤去沉淀，调 pH 5 ~6，加 3% 氯化钙溶液 2 ~3 滴，放置 10 分钟，不得出现浑浊或沉淀。

(5) 重金属 取本品 1.0g，缓缓炽灼至完全炭化，放冷，加硫酸 0.5 ~ 1.0ml，使恰湿润，用低温加热至硫酸除尽后，加硝酸 0.5ml，蒸干，至氧化氮蒸气除尽后，放冷，在 500 ~600℃ 炽灼使完全灰化，放冷，加盐酸 2ml，置水浴上蒸干后加水 15ml，滴加氨试液至对酚酞指示液显中性，再加醋酸盐缓冲液（pH 3.5）2ml，微热溶解后，移至纳氏比色管中，加水稀释成 25ml（乙管）。另取配制供试品溶液的试剂，置瓷皿中蒸干后，加醋酸盐缓冲液（pH 3.5）2ml 与水 15ml，微热溶解后，移至纳氏比色管中，加标准铅溶液一定量，再用水稀释成 25ml（甲管）。在甲乙两管中分别加硫代乙酰胺试液各 2ml，摇匀，放置 2 分钟，同置白纸上，自上向下透视，乙管中显出的颜色与甲管比较，不得更深。

(6) 砷盐 取本品 1.0g，加 2% 硝酸镁乙醇溶液 3ml，点燃，燃尽后，先用小火炽灼使炭化，再在 500 ~600℃ 炽灼使完全灰化，放冷，加盐酸 5ml 与水 21ml 使溶解，照标准砷斑的制备，自 "再加碘化钾试液 5ml" 起，依法操作，将生成的砷斑与标准砷斑比较，不得更深。

标准砷斑的制备：精密量取标准砷溶液 2ml，置 A 瓶中，加盐酸 5ml 与水 21ml，再加碘化钾试液 5ml 与酸性氯化亚锡试液 5 滴，在室温放置 10 分钟后，加锌粒 2g，立即将装妥的导气管 C 密塞于 A 瓶上（见实验四，图 5 - 3），并将 A 瓶置 25 ~40℃ 水浴中，反应 45 分钟，取出溴化汞试纸，即得。

(7) 钾离子 精密称取本品 0.12g，先用小火炽灼至炭化，再在 500 ~600℃ 炽灼至完全灰化，加稀醋酸使溶解，置 25ml 量瓶中，加水稀释至刻度，混匀，作为供试品溶液。取 10ml 纳氏比色管两支，甲管中精密加入标准钾离子溶液 0.8ml，加碱性甲醛溶液（取甲醛溶液，用 0.1mol/L 氢氧化钠调节 pH 至 8.0 ~9.0）12 滴、3% 乙二胺四醋酸二钠溶液 2 滴、3% 四苯硼钠溶液 0.5ml，加水稀释成 10ml。乙管中精密加入供试品溶液 1ml，与甲管同时依法操作，摇匀。甲、乙两管同置黑纸上，自上向下透视，乙管中显出的浊度与甲管比较，不得更浓。

3. 含量测定

(1) 绿原酸的测定

1）色谱条件与系统适用性试验 用十八烷基硅烷键合硅胶为填充剂；甲醇 - 水 - 冰醋酸 - 三乙胺（15∶85∶1∶0.3）为流动相；检测波长为 324nm。理论板数按绿原酸峰计算应不低于 6000。

2）对照溶液的制备 取绿原酸对照品适量，精密称定，加水制成每 1ml 含 0.02mg 的溶液，即得。

3）供试品溶液的制备 取本品装量差异项下的内容物，混匀，取 60mg，精密称定，置 50ml 量瓶中，用水溶解并稀释至刻度，摇匀，即得。

4）测定法　分别精密吸取对照品溶液与供试品溶液各 20μl，注入液相色谱仪，测定，测得峰面积，采用外标一点法，计算样品中黄芩苷的含量，即得。

本品每支含金银花以绿原酸（$C_{16}H_{18}O_9$）计，应为 8.5～11.5mg。

（2）黄芩苷的测定

1）色谱条件与系统适用性试验　色谱柱用十八烷基硅烷键合硅胶为填充剂；甲醇－水－冰醋酸（45:55:1）为流动相；检测波长为 274nm。理论板数按黄芩苷峰计算应不低于 2000。

2）对照品溶液的制备　取黄芩苷对照品适量，精密称定，加 50% 甲醇制成每 1ml 含 0.05mg 的溶液，即得。

3）供试品溶液的制备　取本品装量差异项下的内容物，混匀，取 10mg，精密称定，加 50% 甲醇适量，超声处理 20 分钟使溶解，制成每 1ml 约含 0.2mg 溶液，即得。

4）测定法　精密吸取对照品溶液与供试品溶液各 20μl，注入液相色谱仪，测定，测得峰面积，采用外标一点法，计算样品中黄芩苷的含量，即得。

本品每支含黄芩按黄芩苷（$C_{21}H_{18}O_{11}$）计，应为 128～173mg。

【实验记录】

1. 记录注射用双黄连（冻干）的鉴别实验结果，绘制薄层色谱图并算出主要斑点的 R_f 值。

2. 记录注射用双黄连（冻干）的检查实验结果。

3. 记录含量测定实验数据，分别计算绿原酸和黄芩苷的含量。

【思考题】

1. 鉴别黄芩时为什么可用聚酰胺薄膜色谱？

2. 说明测定黄芩苷含量时流动相中加入冰醋酸的目的。

3. 注射剂中杂质检查项目主要有哪些？

【相关资料】

1. **注射用双黄连（冻干）**　处方：连翘、金银花、黄芩。制法：以上三味，黄芩加水煎煮两次，每次 1 小时，滤过，合并滤液，用 2mol/L 盐酸溶液调节 pH 至 1.0～2.0，在 80℃ 保温 30 分钟，静置 12 小时，滤过，沉淀加 8 倍量水，搅拌，用 40% 氢氧化钠溶液调节 pH 至 6.0～7.0，加入等量乙醇，搅拌使溶解，滤过，滤液用 2mol/L 盐酸溶液调节 pH 至 2.0，在 80℃ 保温 30 分钟，静置 12 小时，滤过，沉淀用乙醇洗至 pH4.0，加适量水，搅拌，用 40% 氢氧化钠溶液调节 pH 至 6.0～7.0，加入适量的活性炭，充分搅拌，在 50℃ 保温 30 分钟，加入 1～2 倍量乙醇，充分搅拌，滤过，滤液用 2mol/L 盐酸溶液调节 pH 至 2.0，在 80℃ 保温 30 分钟，静置 12 小时，滤过，沉淀用少量乙醇洗涤，于 60℃ 以下干燥，备用；金银花、连翘加水温浸 30 分钟，煎煮两次，每次 1 小时，滤过，合并滤液，浓缩至相对密度为 1.20～1.25（70～80℃），放冷至 40℃，缓缓加入乙醇使含醇量达 75%，充分搅拌，静置 12 小时以上，滤取上清液，回收乙醇至无醇味，备用；取黄芩提取物，加入适量的水，加热，用 40% 氢氧化钠溶液调节 pH 至 7.0 使溶解，加入上述金银花、连翘提取物，加水至 1000ml，加入适量的活性炭，调节 pH 至 7.0，加热至沸，并保持微沸 15 分钟，冷却，滤过，加注射用水至全量，灭菌，冷藏，滤过，浓缩，冻干，制成粉末，分装，即得。功能与主治：疏风解表，清热解毒。用于外感风热所致的感冒，症见发热、咳嗽、咽痛。

2. **黄芩** 为唇形科植物黄芩 *Scutellaria baicalensis* Georgi 的干燥根。主要含有黄芩苷（baicalin）、黄芩苷元（baicalein）、汉黄芩素（wogonin）、汉黄芩苷（wogonoside）等三十余种黄酮类化合物。其中黄芩苷为主要有效成分，对照品易得，可作为鉴别和含量测定的依据。

3. **金银花** 为忍冬科植物忍冬 *Lonicera japonica* Thunb.、红腺忍冬 *Lonicera hypoglauca* Miq.、山银花 *Lonicera confusa* DC. 或毛花柱忍冬 *Lonicera dasystyla* Rehd. 的干燥花蕾或带初开的花。主要含有绿原酸（chlorogenic acid）、木犀草素（luteolin）、肌醇（inositol）、异绿原酸（isochlorogenic acid）以及挥发油。绿原酸为金银花的代表成分，可作为鉴别和含量测定的依据。

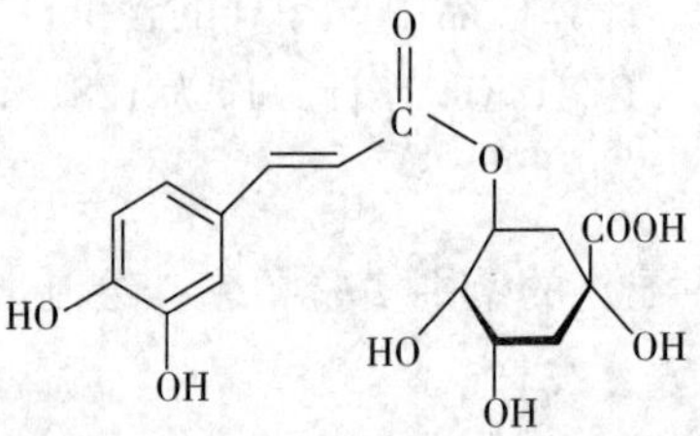

绿原酸

4. **连翘** 为木犀科植物连翘 *Forsythia suspense*（Thunb.）Vahl. 的干燥果实。主要含有连翘酯苷（forsythoside）A、B、C 和 D、连翘酚（forsythol）、连翘苷（phillyrin）、连翘苷元（phillygenin）、齐墩果酸（oleanolic acid）和熊果酸（ursolic acid）等。

5. **黄芩苷** 结构中由于含有一个葡萄糖醛酸，显弱酸性，在流动相中加入了一定比例的冰醋酸，抑制被测成分解离，改善峰形，谱图上各色谱峰的分离较好，黄芩苷的保留时间适中。

6. **试剂的配制**

（1）鞣酸试液 取鞣酸 1g，加乙醇 1ml，加水溶解并稀释至 100ml，即得。本液应临用新制。

（2）氯化钠明胶试液 取白明胶 1g 与氯化钠 10g，加水 100ml，置不超过 60℃ 的水浴上微热使溶解。本液应临用新制。

（3）酚酞指示液 取酚酞 1g，加乙醇 100ml，使溶解，即得。变色范围 8.3~10（无色~红色）。

（4）醋酸盐缓冲液（pH 3.5） 取醋酸铵 25g，加水 25ml 溶解后，加 7mol/L 盐酸溶液 38ml，用 2mol/L 盐酸溶液或 5mol/L 氨溶液准确调 pH 至 3.5（电位法指示），用水稀释至 1000ml，即得。

（5）标准钾离子溶液 取硫酸钾适量，研细，于 110℃ 干燥至恒重，精密称取 2.330g，置 1000ml 量瓶中，加水适量使溶解并稀释至刻度，摇匀，作为贮备液。临用前，精密量取贮备液 10ml，置 100ml 量瓶中，加水稀释至刻度，摇匀，即得。（每 1ml 相当于 100μg 的钾）。

（6）标准砷溶液 称取三氧化二砷 0.132g，置 1000ml 量瓶中，加入 20% 氢氧化钠溶液 5ml 溶解后，用适量的稀硫酸中和，再加稀硫酸 10ml，用水稀释至刻度，摇匀，作为贮备液。临用前，精密取贮备液 10ml，置 1000ml 量瓶中，加稀硫酸 10 毫升，用水稀释至刻度，摇匀，即得（每 1ml 相当于 1μg 的砷）。

（7）标准铅溶液 称取硝酸铅 0.160g，置 1000ml 量瓶中，加硝酸 5ml 与水 50ml 溶解后，用水稀释至刻度，摇匀，作为贮备液。临用前，精密取贮备液 10ml，置 1000ml 量瓶中，加水稀释至刻度，摇匀，即得（每 1ml 相当于 1μg 的铅）。配制与贮存用的玻璃容器均不得含铅。

（8）碱性甲醛溶液 取甲醛溶液，用 0.1mol/L 氢氧化钠调节 pH 至 8.0~9.0。

（9）3% 四苯硼钠溶液 取四苯硼钠 31g，加水 215ml 使溶解加入新配制的氢氧化铝凝胶（取三氯化铝 4.0g，溶于 100ml 水中，在不断搅拌下缓缓滴加氢氧化钠试剂至 pH 8~9），加氯化钠 71.1g，充分摇匀。加水 250ml，振摇 15 分钟，静置 10 分钟，滤过，滤液中滴加氢氧化钠试剂至 pH 8~9，再加水稀释至 1000ml，摇匀。

（10）碘化钾试液 取碘化钾 16.5g，加水使溶解成 100ml，即得，本液应临用新制。

（11）硫代乙酰胺试液 取硫代乙酰胺 4g，加水使溶解成 100ml，至冰箱中保存，临用前取混合液（由 1mol/L 氢氧化钠溶液 15ml，水 5.0ml 及甘油 20ml 组成）5.0ml，加上述硫代乙酰胺溶液 1.0ml，置水浴上加热 20 秒，冷却立即使用。

（12）酸性氯化亚锡试液 取氯化亚锡 20g，加盐酸使溶解成 50ml，滤过即得。本液配成后 3 个月即不适用。

Experiment 16　Quality Analysis of Shuanghuanglian for Oral Liquid

Purpose

1. To master the determination of effective components of Traditional Chinese patent medicine by HPLC.

2. To master the purpose and principle and operational method in the test for foreign matter of injection.

Principle

Thin layer chromatography is used to identifytraditional Traditional Chinese patent medicines in comparison with reference substances and reference drugs. The test items of foreign matter about injection mainly include: the test for protein (the test of adding tannic acid), tannin (the test of adding albumen or sodium chloride and galatin TS), the limit test for heavy metals (the test of complying with the method in Chinese Pharmacopoeia, not more than 0.001%), the limit test for arsenic (the test of complying with the method in Chinese Pharmacopoeia, not more than 0.0002%), the test for oxalate (the test of adding calcium chloride), the test for potassium iron (test by sodium tetraphenylborate), the test for resin (the test of adding hydrochloric acid or glacial acetic acid). High performance liquid chromatography is used to determine the content of chlorogenic acid or baicalin, and the maximum absorbent wavelength of chlorogenic acid or baicalin is selected as the wavelength of the detector.

Apparatus, Materials and Reagents

1. Apparatus: high performance liquid chromatogram, ultrasonic surge, ultraviolet light, muffle furnace.

2. Materials: silica gel G – TLC plate (5 cm × 10 cm), polyamide film (5 cm × 7.5 cm), vertical developing chamber (10 cm × 10 cm), volumetric flask (25 ml), Nessler cylinder, capillaries, test tube, filter paper, funnel, separate funnel.

3. Reagents: methanol (chromatographically pure), 75% methanol (analytically pure), glacial acetic acid, chloroform, distilled water, 10% sulfuric acid in ethanol solution, tannic acid TS, dilute acetic acid, sodium chloride and galatin TS, hydrochloric acid, dilute sodium hydroxide, 3% calcium chloride solution, phenolphthalein IS, acetate BS (pH 3.5), potassium iron standard solution, standard arsenic solution, standard lead solution, alkaline formaldehyde, 3% disodium edetate solution, 3% sodium tetraphenylborate solution, triethylamine;

4. Drugs: baicalin CRS 75% methanol solution (0.1 mg/ml), baicalin CRS 50% methanol solution (0.05 mg/ml), chlorogenic acid CRS 75% methanol solution (0.1 mg/ml), chlorogenic acid CRS 75% water solution (0.02 mg/ml); Fructus Forsythiae reference drug solution (dissolve 0.5 g in 5 ml of methanol, ultrasonicate for 20 minutes); Shuanghuanglian for injection (for sale).

Experiment contents

1. Identification

(1) Identification of Scutellariae Radix and Lonicerae Japonicae Flos　To 60 mg, add 3 ml of 75% methanol, ultrasonicate to dissolve as the test solution, take 0.1 g of Scutellariae Radix and 0.2 g of Forsythiae Fructus respectively, add 5 ml of 75% methanol, ultrasonicate for 10 minutes as the negative reference solution of Lonicerae Japonicae Flos; take 0.1 g of Lonicerae Japonicae Flos and 0.2 g of Forsythiae Fructus respectively, add 5 ml of 75% methanol, ultrasonicate for 10 minutes as the negative reference solution of Scutellariae Radix; using acetic acid as the mobile phase, apply separately of each of the three above solutions and baicalin CRS 75% methanol solution, chlorogenic acid CRS 75% methanol solution to a polyamide film 1 μl, after developing and removal of the film, dry it in air, examine under ultraviolet light (365 nm). The fluorescent spots in the chromatogram obtained with the test solution correspond in position and colour to the spots in the chromatogram obtained with the reference solution.

(2) Identification of Forsythiae Fructus　To 0.1 g, add 5 ml of methanol, ultrasonicate for 20 minutes, and allow to stand, using the supernatant as the test solution, using silica gel G containing sodium carboxymethylcellulose as the coating substance and chloroform – methanol

(20:1) as the mobile phase, apply separately of each of Fructus Forsythiae reference drug solution and the test solution to the plate 10 μl, after developing and removal of the plate, dry it in air, spray with a solution of 10% sulfuric acid in ethanol sollution, heat at 100 ℃ until spots distinct. The spots in the chromatogram obtained with the test solution correspond in position and colour to the spots in the chromatogram obtained with the reference drug solution.

2. Test

(1) Protein　Transfer 0. 1 g into a test tube, add 2 ml of water, ultrasonicate to dissolve, add 1 – 3 drops of tannic acid TS, no opalescence is produced.

(2) Tannin　Transfer 0. 1 g into a test tube, add 2 ml of water, ultrasonicate to dissolve, add 1 drop of dilute acetic acid, then add 4 – 5 drops of sodium chloride and galatin TS, no opalescence or precipitate is produced.

(3) Resin　Take 0. 3 g into a test tube, dissolve it in 5 ml of water and transfer it into a separating funnel, add 10 ml of chloroform, shake well, separate the chloroform solution, evaporate on a water bath to dry, add 2 ml of glacial acetic acid in the residue to dissolve it, then pour into a test tube with plug, add 3 ml of water and mix well, allow to stand for 30 minutes, no flocculus should appear.

(4) Oxalate　Transfer 0. 1 g into a test tube, add 2 ml of water, ultrasonicate to dissolve, adjust to pH 1 – 2 with dilute hydrochloric acid, then fliter, adjust the filtrate to pH 5 – 6, add 2 – 3 drops of 3% calcium chloride solution, allow to stand for 10 minutes, no opalescence or precipitate is produced.

(5) Heavy metals　Ignite 1. 0 g of the sample in a crucible until thoroughly charred, cool, moisten the residue with 0. 5 – 1. 0 ml of sulfuric acid, ignite at a low temperature until sulfurous acid fumes are no longer evolved, add 0. 5 ml of nitric acid, evaporate to dryness, heat until nitrous oxide fumes are no longer evolved and ignite at 500 – 600 ℃ until the incineration is complete, cool, add 2 ml of hydrochloric acid, evaporate to dryness on a water bath, add 15 ml of water, followed by ammonia TS dropwise until the solution is neutral to phenolphthalein IS, then add 2 ml of acetate BS (pH 3. 5) and warm to effect dissolution, transfer the resulting solution to Nessler cylinder B, dilute with water to 25 ml. Place the same quantity of the same reagents used for the preparation of test solution in a porcelain dish and evaporate to dryness, heat gently to dissolve in 2 ml of acetate BS (pH 3. 5) and 15 ml of water, transfer to the Nessler cylinder A and add the specified volume of standard lead solution, dilute with water to 25 ml. To each cylinder, add 2 ml of thioacetamide TS and mix well, allow to stand for 2 minutes, compare the colour produced by viewing down the vertical axis of the cylinders against a white background, the colour produced in cylinder B is not more intense than that produced in cylinder A.

(6) Arsenic　To 1. 0 g, add 3 ml of solution of 2% magnesium nitrate in ethanol, fire to burn, after burning out, heat gently until it is charred, then ignite at 500 – 600 ℃ until incineration is completed, allow to cool, dissolve in 5 ml of hydrochloric acid and 21 ml of water,

proceed as described under arsenic standard stain beginning with the words "Then add 5 ml of potassium iodide TS···", and stain produced is not more intense than the standard stain.

Arsenic standard stain: Place 2 ml of standard arsenic solution, accurately measured, in flask A, add 5 ml of hydrochloric acid and 21 ml of water, then add 5 ml of potassium iodide TS and 5 drops of acid stannous chloride TS, allow to stand at room temperature for 10 minutes and add 2 g of zinc granules, insert the stopper B and conduit C into the mouth of flask A and immerse the flask in a water bath at 25 – 40 ℃ for 45 minutes, remove the mercuric bromide test paper. (Experiment 4 Figure 2 – 3)

(7) Potassium iron   Weigh 0. 12 g accurately, first, ignite till carbonized with weak flame, then incinerate at 500 – 600℃ until carbon – free, add dilute acetic acid to dissolve, and transfer into 25 ml volumetric flask, dilute with water to the volume and mix well, use as a test solution. Take two Nessler cylinder, measure accurately potassium iron standard solution 0. 8 ml in tube A, add 12 drops of alkaline formaldehyde (measure formaldehyde solution, adjust the pH value to 8. 0 – 9. 0 with sodium hydroxide), 2 drops of 3% disodium edetate solution, 0. 5 ml of 3% sodium tetraphenylborate solution, dilute with water to 10 ml. Measure accurately 1 ml of the test solution in tube B, process as what done on tube A at the same time, shake well. Compare to opalescence produced by viewing down the vertical axis of the cylinders against a black background, opalescence of tube B should not be heavier than that of tube A. (Experiment 4 Figure 2 – 3)

3. Assay

(1) Determination of chlorogenic acid

Chromatographic system and system suitability: Use octadecylsilane bonded silica gel as the stationary phase and methanol – water – glacial acetic acid – triethylamine (15:85:1:0. 3) as the mobile phase; the wavelength of the detector is 324 nm. The number of theoretical plates of the column is not less than 6000, calculated with reference to the peak of chlorogenic acid.

Preparation of reference solution: Dissolve a quantity of chlorogenic acid CRS, weighed accurately, in water to produce a solution containing 0. 02 mg per ml.

Preparation of test solution: Mix the contents obtained in the test of weight variation, weigh accurately 60 mg to a 50 ml volumetric flask, dissolve and dilute to volume with water, and mix well, used as the test solution.

Procedure: Accurately inject 20 μl of each of the reference solution and the test solution respectively, into the column, determine the peak area, use the external standard one – point method to calculate the content of baicalin in the sample.

It contains not less than 8. 5 mg and not more than 11. 5 mg chlorogenic acid ($C_{16}H_{18}O_9$) per vial referred to Lonicerae Japonicae Flos.

(2) Determine of Baicalin

Chromatographic system and system suitability: Use octadecylsilane boned silica gel as the stationary phase and methanol – water – glacial acid (45:55:1) as the mobile phase; the wavelength of the detector is 274 nm. The number of theoretical plates of the column is not less than 2000, calculated with reference to the peak of baicalin.

Preparation of reference solution: Dissolve a quantity of Baicalin CRS, weighed accurately, in 50% methanol to produce a solution containing 0.05 mg per ml as the reference solution.

Preparation of test solution: Mix the contents obtained in the test of weight variation, weigh accurately 10 mg, add a quantity of 50% methanol, ultrasonicate for 20 minutes to dissolve, to produce a solution containing about 0.2 mg per ml as the reference solution.

Procedure: Accurately inject 20 μl of each of the reference solution and the test solution respectively, into the column, determine the peak area, use the external standard one – point method to calculate the content of baicalin in the sample.

It contains not less than 128 mg and not more than 173 mg of baicalin ($C_{21}H_{18}O_{11}$) per vial, referred to Scutellariae Radix.

Experiment records

1. Record the TLC identification test, plot the TLC chromatograms and calculate the R_f value of major spots.

2. Record the test of foreign matter.

3. Record the assay data and calculate the content of chlorogenic acid and baicalin respectively.

Questions

1. Why can we use the polyamide film for chromatography in the identification of Scutellariae Radix?

2. Explain the purpose of adding glacial acetic acid in the mobile phase when determining the content of baicalin?

3. What are the main test items of foreign matter about injection?

Related materials

1. Ingredients of Shuanghuanglian for injection: Forsythiae Fructus, Lonicerae Japonicae Flos, and Scutellariae Radix. Procedure: decoct Scutellariae Radix with water for two times, one hour for each, filter, combine the filtrate, and adjust to pH 1.0 – 2.0 with 2 mol/L solution of hydrochloric acid. Allow to keep warm at 80 ℃ for 30 minutes, and stand for 12 hours. Filter, stir the precipitate with 8 volume of water, adjust to pH 6.0 – 7.0 with 40% solution of sodium hydroxide, add equal quantities of ethanol, stir to dissolve, and filter. To the filtrate adjust to pH 2.0, keep warm at 80 ℃ for 30 minutes, and stand for 12 hours, and filter. Wash the precipitate with ethanol to pH 4.0, add a quantity of water, stir, and adjust to pH 6.0 – 7.0. Add a quantity of activated charcoal, stir thoroughly, keep warm at 50 ℃ for 30 minutes, add 1 to 2 volume of ethanol and stir well. Filter, adjust the filtrate to pH 2.0 with 2 mol/L solution of hydrochloric acid, keep warm at 80 ℃ for 30 minutes, and stand for 12 hours. Filter, wash the precipitate with small quantities of ethanol, dry below 60 ℃ for further use. Macerate Lonicerae Japonicae Flos and Forsythiae Fructus with water for 30 minutes, de-

coct for two times, one hour for each, and filter. Combine the filtrates, concentrate to a thick extract of relative density of 1. 20 – 1. 25 (70 – 80 ℃), allow to stand to 40℃, and add slowly ethanol to make the content to 75% ethanol, and stir thoroughly. Stand for 12 hours, filter and recover solvent to ethanol odorless. To extract of Scutellariae Radix add a quantity of water, heat and dissolve by adjusting to pH 7. 0 with 40% solution of sodium hydroxide. Mix with the above extract of Lonicerae Japonicae Flos and Forsythiae Fructus, add water to 1000 ml, add a quantity of activated charcoal, adjust to pH 7. 0, heat to boil and keep boiling for 15 minutes. Stand to cool, filter, add water for injection to total volume, sterile, refrigerate, filter, concentrate, freeze to powder and pack. Action: To clear heat to relieve toxicity, and disperse wind to release the exterior. Indications: fever, coughing and sore throat due to affliction from exogenous wind – heat; upper respiratory tract infection, mild pneumonia or tonsillitis with above symptoms.

2. Scutellariae Radix is the dried roots of *Scutellaria baicalensis* Georgi. It mainly contains flavonoids including baicalin, baicalein, wogonin, wogonoside etc. , Among the flavonoids, baicalin is the main active constituent and also available, so it is usually selected as reference substance in identification and determination.

3. Lonicerae Japonicae Flos is the blossom bud of *Lonicera japonica* Thunb. , *Lonicera hypoglauca* Miq. , *Lonicera confusa* DC. , or *Lonicera dasystyla* Rehd. It mainly contains chlorogenic acid, luteolin, inositol, isochlorogenic acid, and volatile oil. Chlorogenic acid is its main active constituent.

chlorogenic acid

4. Forsythiae Fructus is the dried fruits of *Forsythia suspense* (Thunb.) Vahl. It contains many lignans such as forsythoside A, B, C, D and forsythol, phillyrin, phillygenin etc.

5. As the structure of baicalin contains a glucuronic – acid unit, it is faintly acid, add certainly proportional glacial acetic acid inthe mobile phase, the peaks in the chromatogram separate well and the retention time of baicalin is moderate.

6. The preparation of reagents

(1) Tannic acid TS   Dissolve 1 g of tannic acid in 1 ml of alcohol and dilute with water to 100 ml. This solution should be freshly prepared.

(2) Sodium chloride and galatin TS   Dissolve 1 g of gelatin and 10 g of sodium chloride in 100 ml of water by heat on a water bath at a temperature below 60 ℃.

(3) Phenolphthalein IS   Dissolve 1 g of phenolphthalein in 100 ml of ethanol. Colour

changes from colourless to red (pH 8. 3 – 10. 0).

(4) Acetate BS (pH 3. 5)　Dissolve 25g of ammonium acetate in 25 ml of water, add 38 ml of hydrochloric acid solution (7 mol/L) . Adopt the potentiometric acid solution (2 mol/L) or ammonia solution (5 mol/L) and dilute with water to 1000 ml.

(5) Potassium iron standard solution　Place suitable potassium sulfate, grind into fine power, dry to constant weigh at 110 ℃, weigh 2. 330 g accurately, put into 1000 ml volumetric flask, add sufficient water to dissolve and dilute to the volume, shake well, use as store solution. Immediately before using, measure accurately the store solution 10 ml in 100 ml volumetric flask, dilute with water to volume and shake well (each ml equals to 100 μg of potassium) .

(6) Standard arsenic solution　Dissolve 0. 132 g of arsenic trioxide with 5 ml of 20% sodium hydroxide solution in a 1000 ml volumetric flask, neutralize with dilute sulfuric acid and add 10 ml in excess, dilute with water to the volume and mix well , as a stock solution. Transfer 10 ml of the stock solution, accurately measured, to a 1000 ml volumetric flask immediately before use, add 10 ml of dilute sulfuric acid, dilute with water to the volume and mix well (each ml is equivalent to 1 μg of As).

(7) Standard lead solution　Dissolve 0. 160 g of lead nitrate with 5 ml of nitric acid and 50 ml of water in a 1000 ml volumetric flask, dilute to volume with water, mix well (stock solution) . Transfer 10 ml of the stock solution, accurately measured, to a 1000 ml volumetric flask, dilute with water to the volume and mix well (each ml is equivalent to 1 μg of Pb). This solution should be prepared immediately before use. All glassware used for the preparation and preservation of standard lead solution should be free from lead.

(8) Alkaline formaldehyde　Measure formaldehyde solution, adjust the pH value to 8. 0 – 9. 0 with sodium hydroxide (0. 1mol/L).

(9) 3% sodium tetraphenylborate solution　Dissolve 31 g of sodium tetraphenylborate in 215 ml of water with shake. Add freshly prepared aluminum hydroxide gel (dissolve 4. 0 g of aluminum chloride in 100 ml of water, add sodium hydroxide TS dropwise with stirring until the pH is 8 – 9), 71. 1 g of sodium chloride and stir thoroughly. Add 250 ml of water and shake for 15 minutes, allow to stand for 10 minutes and filter. Add sodium hydroxide TS dropwise to the filtrate until the pH is 8 – 9, and then dilute with water to 1000 ml, mix well.

(10) Potassium Iodide TS　Dissolve 16. 5 g of potassium iodide in water to make 100 ml. This solution should be freshly prepared.

(11) Thioacetamide TS　Dissolve 4 g of thioacetamide in water to make 100 ml. Store in refrigerator. Add 1. 0 ml of thioacetamide solution to 5. 0 ml of a mixture consisting of 15 ml sodium hydroxide solution (1 mol/L) , 5. 0 ml of water and 20 ml of glycerin before use, heat for 20 seconds in a water bath, cool and use immediately.

(12) Acid stannous chloride TS　Dissolve 20 g of stannous chloride in hydrochloric acid to make 50 ml and filter.

实验十七　六味地黄丸的质量分析

【目的要求】

1. 熟悉中药制剂质量分析的主要内容。
2. 熟悉中药制剂质量分析的常用方法及操作。

【原理】

六味地黄丸为药材粉末直接入药，保留有原药材的组织、细胞或内含物等显微特征，可以据此采用显微鉴别方法鉴别中药制剂的处方；同时可以利用薄层色谱法鉴别处方。用高效液相色谱法对处方中山茱萸所含马钱苷及牡丹皮中丹皮酚进行含量测定。

【仪器、试剂与药品】

1. **仪器**　高效液相色谱仪、显微镜、超声波清洗器、分析天平、微量进样器、恒温水浴锅。

2. **材料**　载玻片、盖玻片、酒精灯、乳钵、擦镜纸、小镊子、小刀、冷凝管（24#）、圆底烧瓶（24#，250ml）、量瓶、移液管、滤纸、漏斗、蒸发皿、硅胶 G 薄层板（5cm × 10cm）、毛细管、立式展开槽（10cm × 10cm）、具塞锥形瓶、色谱柱（内径 1cm）。

3. **试剂与试药**　中性氧化铝、硅藻土、乙醚、丙酮、环己烷、乙酸乙酯、四氢呋喃、乙腈、甲醇、重蒸水、稀甘油、水合氯醛试液、甘油醋酸试液、盐酸酸性 5% 三氯化铁乙醇溶液、0.05% 磷酸溶液、50% 甲醇溶液、40% 甲醇溶液。

4. **药品**　马钱苷对照品、丹皮酚对照品（中国食品药品检定研究院）；六味地黄丸（市售品）。

【实验内容】

1. **显微鉴别**　取本品 1 丸，切碎，120℃干燥 2 小时，放冷至室温，粉碎至细粉，取少许细粉，先用甘油醋酸试液装片，置显微镜下观察。再取少许细粉，用水合氯醛试液透化后滴加适量稀甘油，置显微镜下观察。

2. **牡丹皮的鉴别**　取本品水蜜丸6g，研细；或取小蜜丸或大蜜丸9g，剪碎，加硅藻土4g，研匀。加乙醚40ml，回流 1 小时，滤过，滤液挥去乙醚，残渣加丙酮1ml使溶解，作为供试品溶液。另取丹皮酚对照品，加丙酮制成每1ml含1mg的溶液，作为对照品溶液。吸取上述两种溶液各 10 µl，分别点于同一硅胶 G 薄层板上，以环己烷 - 乙酸乙酯（3∶1）为展开剂，展开，取出，晾干，喷以盐酸酸性 5% 三氯化铁乙醇溶液，在 105℃加热数分钟至斑点显色清晰。供试品色谱中，在与对照品色谱相应的位置上，显相同的蓝褐色斑点。

3. 含量测定

（1）山茱萸中马钱苷的测定

1）色谱条件与系统适用性试验 以十八烷基硅烷键合硅胶为填充剂；四氢呋喃 – 乙腈 – 甲醇 – 0.05% 磷酸溶液（1:8:4:87）为流动相；检测波长为 236nm；柱温 40℃。理论板数按马钱苷峰计算应不低于 4000。

2）对照品溶液的制备 取马钱苷对照品适量，精密称定，加 50% 甲醇制成每 1ml 含 20μg 的溶液，即得。

3）供试品溶液的制备 取本品水蜜丸或小蜜丸，切碎，取约 0.7g，精密称定；或取重量差异项下的大蜜丸，剪碎，取约 1g，精密称定，置具塞锥形瓶中，精密加入 50% 甲醇 25ml，密塞，称定重量，超声处理（功率 250W，频率 33kHz）15 分钟使溶散，加热回流 1 小时，放冷，再称定重量，用 50% 甲醇补足减失的重量，摇匀，滤过。精密量取续滤液 10ml，置中性氧化铝柱（100 ~ 200 目，4g，内径 1cm，干法装柱）上，用 40% 甲醇 50ml 洗脱，收集流出液及洗脱液，蒸干，残渣加 50% 甲醇适量溶解，并转移至 10ml 量瓶中，加 50% 甲醇稀释至刻度，摇匀，即得。

4）测定法 分别精密吸取对照品溶液与供试品溶液各 10μl，注入液相色谱仪，测定，测得峰面积，采用外标一点法，计算样品中马钱苷的含量，即得。

本品含山茱萸以马钱苷（$C_{17}H_{26}O_{10}$）计，水蜜丸每 1g 不得少于 0.70mg；小蜜丸每 1g 不得少于 0.50mg；大蜜丸每丸不得少于 4.5mg。

（2）牡丹皮中丹皮酚的测定

1）色谱条件与系统适用性试验 以十八烷基硅烷键合硅胶为填充剂；甲醇 – 水（70:30）为流动相；检测波长为 274nm。理论板数按丹皮酚峰计算应不低于 3500。

2）对照品溶液的制备 取丹皮酚对照品适量，精密称定，加甲醇制成每 1ml 含 20μg 的溶液，即得。

3）供试品溶液的制备 取本品水蜜丸或小蜜丸，切碎，取约 0.3g，精密称定；或取重量差异项下的大蜜丸，剪碎，取约 0.4g，精密称定，置具塞锥形瓶中，精密加入 50% 甲醇 50ml，密塞，称定重量，超声处理（功率 250W，频率 33kHz）45 分钟，放冷，再称定重量，用 50% 甲醇补足减失的重量，摇匀，滤过，取续滤液，即得。

4）测定法 分别精密吸取对照品溶液 10μl 与供试品溶液 20μl，注入液相色谱仪，测定，测得峰面积，采用外标一点法，计算样品中丹皮酚的含量，即得。

本品含牡丹皮以丹皮酚（$C_9H_{10}O_3$）计，水蜜丸每 1g 不得少于 0.90mg；小蜜丸每 1g 不得少于 0.70mg；大蜜丸每丸不得少于 6.3mg。

【实验记录】

1. 记录六味地黄丸的显微鉴别实验结果，绘制显微鉴别图。

2. 记录六味地黄丸中丹皮酚的薄层鉴别结果，绘制薄层色谱图。

3. 记录含量测定原始数据，计算供试品中马钱苷及丹皮酚的含量。

【思考题】

1. 实验中观察到的显微特征分别为何种中药材的特征？

2. 实验中有哪些注意事项？

【相关资料】

1. **六味地黄丸**　处方：熟地黄 160g，山茱萸（制）80g，牡丹皮 60g，山药 80g，茯苓 60g，泽泻 60g。制法：以上六味，粉碎成细粉，过筛，混匀。每 100g 粉末加炼蜜 35～50g 与适量的水，泛丸，干燥，制成水蜜丸；或加炼蜜 80～110g 制成小蜜丸或大蜜丸，即得。功能与主治：滋阴补肾。用于肾阴亏损，头晕耳鸣，腰膝酸软，骨蒸潮热，盗汗遗精，消渴。

熟地黄为玄参科植物地黄 *Rehmannia glutinosa* Libosch. 的新鲜或干燥块根的炮制加工品。主要含环烯醚萜类化合物，如梓醇。山茱萸为山茱萸科植物山茱萸 *Cornus officinalis* Sieb. et Zucc. 的干燥成熟果肉。含马钱苷、熊果酸等。牡丹皮为毛茛科植物牡丹 *Paeonia suffruticosa* Andr. 的干燥根皮。含丹皮酚、芍药苷、挥发油等。山药为薯蓣科植物薯蓣 *Dioscorea opposita* Thunb. 的干燥根茎。主要含淀粉、黏液质，如甘露聚糖和植酸。茯苓为多孔菌科真菌茯苓 *Poria cocos*（Schw.）Wolf 的干燥菌核。含 β-茯苓聚糖、茯苓酸、齿孔酸、块苓酸、松苓酸等。泽泻为泽泻科植物泽泻 *Alisma orientalis*（Sam.）Juzep. 的干燥块茎。主要含四环三萜衍生物，如泽泻醇 A、B、C。

处方中君药熟地黄滋养肾阴、益精；山茱萸和山药为臣药，山茱萸养血，滋养肝阴、肾阴，涩精；山药益气，养脾阴，固精。以上三味分别滋养肾、肝、脾阴。牡丹皮泻肝火，清热凉血；茯苓燥脾湿，助山药益气养脾；泽泻泻肾火、祛湿邪，纠正熟地黄滋腻之性。以上三味为佐使药。此方特点为"三补三泻"，因此质量控制也应在中医理论指导下进行。

2. **显微鉴别实验**　观察淀粉粒和不规则分枝状团块应使用甘油醋酸试液装片，其余特征用水合氯醛试液透化后滴加适量稀甘油观察。其中，山药：淀粉粒呈三角状卵形或矩圆形，直径 24～40μm，脐点短缝状或人字形；草酸钙针晶成束存在于黏液细胞中，针晶较粗长；茯苓：不规则分枝状团块无色，遇水合氯醛试液溶化，菌丝无色，直径 4～6μm；熟地黄：薄壁组织灰棕色至黑棕色，细胞多皱缩，内含棕色核状物；牡丹皮：草酸钙簇晶存在于无色薄壁细胞中，有时数个排列成行；山茱萸：果皮表皮细胞橙黄色，表面观类多角形，垂周壁连珠状增厚；泽泻：薄壁细胞类圆形，有椭圆形纹孔，集成纹孔群；内皮层细胞垂周壁波状弯曲，较厚，木化，有稀疏细孔沟。

六味地黄丸的显微鉴别见图 6-2。

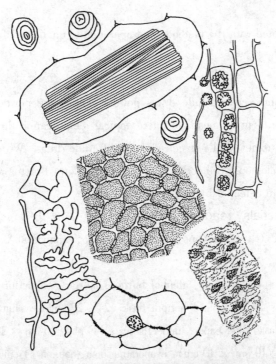

图 6-2 六味地黄丸的显微鉴别图

1. 熟地黄薄壁细胞 2. 山茱萸果皮表皮细胞 3. 牡丹皮草酸钙簇晶 4. 牡丹皮木栓细胞
5. 山药草酸钙针晶 6. 山药淀粉粒 7. 茯苓菌丝 8. 泽泻薄壁细胞

3. 马钱苷和丹皮酚的化学结构式

马钱苷

丹皮酚

4. 试剂的配制

（1）稀甘油 取甘油33ml，加水稀释使成100ml，再加樟脑一小块或液化苯酚1滴，即得。

（2）水合氯醛试液 取水合氯醛50g，加水15ml与甘油10ml使溶解，即得。

（3）甘油醋酸试液 取甘油、50%醋酸与水各等份，混合，即得。

Experiment 17 Quality Analysis of Liuwei Dihuang Pills

Purpose

1. To be familiar with the main contents of quality analysis of Traditional Chinese patent

medicine.

2. To be acquainted with the methods and operation of quality analysis of Traditional Chinese patent medicine.

Principle

As the patent composed of crude drugs powder retains the powder characters of crude drugs, we can identify them by means of microscopical identification through observing microscopical characters of tissues, cells or cell contents of crude drugs. We can also identify drugs in the patent by TLC method. The contents of loganin in Corni Fructus and paeonol in Moutan Cortex in the patent are detected by HPLC method.

Apparatus, materials, reagents and drugs

1. Apparatus: HPLC, microscope, ultrasonic surge, analytical balance, microsyringe, water bath.

2. Materials: slide, cover glass, alcohol burner, mortar, paper for erasing lens, nipper, knife, condenser tube ($24^{\#}$), round bottom flask ($24^{\#}$, 250 ml), volumetric flask, transfer pipette, stopper conical flask, filter paper, funnel, silica gel G plate (5 cm × 10 cm), capillary, vertical developing chamber (10 cm × 10 cm), evaporating dish, column (1 cm in internal diameter).

3. Reagents: neutral aluminum oxide for chromatic spectrum, kieselguhr, ether, acetone, cyclohexane, ethyl acetate, tetrahydrofuran, acetonitrile, methanol (chromatographically pure), redistilled water, glycerin dilute TS, chloral hydrate TS, glycerin – acetic acid TS, 5% solution of ferric chloride in ethanol acidified with hydrochloric acid, 0.05% solution of phosphoric acid, 50% methanol solution, 40% methanol solution.

4. Drugs: loganin CRS, paeonol CRS (provided by National Institute for Food and Drug control); Liuwei Dihuang Pills (for sale).

Experiment contents

1. Microscopical identification of Liuwei Dihuang Pills

Cut 1 pill into pieces and dry for 2 hours at 120 ℃, cool to room temperature and triturate to fine powder. To a small quantity of the powder, use glycerin – acetic acid TS as mountant and observed under the microscope. Others can be observed under the microscope by adding dropwise an adequate quantity of dilute glycerin after the disposal of chloral hydrate TS.

2. Identification of Moutan Cortex

To 9 g of small honeyed pills or big honeyed pills, or 6 g of water – honeyed pills, in powder, add 4 g of ether and triturate well. Heat under reflux with 40 ml of ether at a low temperature for 1 hour, filter and evaporate to remove ether. Dissolve the residue in 1 ml of acetone as the test solution. Dissolve paeonol CRS in acetone to produce a solution containing 1 mg per ml, as the reference solution. Using silica gel G as the coating substance and cyclohexane – ethyl acetate (3:1) as the mobile phase. Apply separately to the plate 10 μl of each of the two solutions. After developing and removal of the plate, dry it in air, spray with 5% solution of ferric chloride in ethanol acidified with hydrochloric acid and visualize under a current of hot air (105 ℃). The bluish – brown spot in the chromatogram obtained with the test solution corresponds in position and colour to the spot in the chromatogram obtained with the reference solution.

3. Assay

(1) Determine of loganin

Chromatographic system and system suitability: Use octadecylsilane bonded silica gel as the stationary phase and tetrahydrofuran – acetonitrile – methanol – 0.05% solution of phosphoric acid (1:8:4:87) as the mobile phase; the wavelength of the detector is 236 nm; column temperature is 40 ℃. The number of theoretical plates of the column is not less than 4000, calculated with reference to the peak of loganin.

Preparation of reference solution: Dissolve a quantity of loganin CRS, weighed accurately, in 50% methanol to produce a solution containing 20 μg per ml.

Preparation of test solution: Cut the water – honeyed pills or the small honeyed pills into pieces, weigh accurately 0.7 g (or cut the big honeyed pills in the test of weigh variation into pieces, weigh accurately 1 g) to a stopper conical flask, accurately add 25 ml of 50% methanol, stopper tightly and weigh, ultrasonicate for 15 minutes (power 250 W, frequency 33 kHz), heat under reflux for 1 hour, allow to cool, weigh again, replenish the loss of the solvent with 50% methanol, mix well, filter and transfer accurately 10 ml successive filtrate into neutral aluminum oxide column (100 – 200 mesh, 4 g, about 1 cm in internal diameter, packed by dry method), elute with 50 ml of 40% methanol in portions, collect the eluent and evaporate to dryness. Dissolve the residue with a suitable quantity of 50% methanol and transfer into a 10 ml volumetric flask, dilute with 50% methanol to volume and mix well.

Procedure: Accurately inject 10 μl of each of the reference solution and the test solution respectively, into the column, determine the peak area, use the external standard one – point method to calculate the content of loganin in the sample.

The big honeyed pillsc ontain not less than 4.5 mg per pills; the water – honeyed pills and the small honeyed pills contain not less than 0.70 mg and 0.50 mg per gram of loganin ($C_{17}H_{26}O_{10}$), referred to Corni Fructus.

(2) Determine of paeonol

Chromatographic system and system suitability: Use octadecylsilane bonded silica gel as the stationary phase and methanol – water (70:30) as the mobile phase; the wavelength of the detector is 274 nm. The number of theoretical plates of the column is not less than 3500, calculated with reference to the peak of paeonol.

Preparation of reference solution: Dissolve a quantity of paeonol CRS, weighed accurately, in methanol to produce a solution containing 20 μg per ml.

Preparation of test solution: Cut the water – honeyed pills or the small honeyed pills into pieces, weigh accurately 0. 3 g (or cut the big honeyed pills in the test of weigh variation into pieces, weigh accurately 0. 4 g) to a stopper conical flask, accurately add 50 ml of 50% methanol, stopper tightly and weigh, ultrasonicate for 45 minutes (power 250 W, frequency 33 kHz), allow to cool, weigh again, replenish the loss of the solvent with 50% methanol, mix well, filter and use the successive filtrate.

Procedure: Accurately inject 10 μl of the reference solution and 20 μl of the test solution respectively, into the column, determine the peak area, use the external standard one – point method to calculate the content of paeonol in the sample.

The big honeyed pills contain not less than 6. 3 mg per pills; the water – honeyed pills and the small honeyed pills contain not less than 0. 90 mg and 0. 70 mg per gram of paeonol ($C_9H_{10}O_3$), referred to Cortex Moutan.

Experiment records

1. Record the microscopic identification test result of Liuwei Dihuang Pills and draw the micrograph.

2. Record the TLC identification test result of Moutan Cortex and draw the TLC chromatogram.

3. Record the original data of content test and calculate the content of loganin and paeonol in sample.

Questions

1. Try to describe the microscopical characters you observed, which traditional Chinese drugs dose each of them stand for?

2. What must we pay more attention to during the operation procedure?

Related materials

1. Ingredients of Liuwei Dihuang Pills: Rehmanniae Radix Preparata 160 g, Corni Fructus (processed with wine) 80 g, Moutan Cortex 60 g, Dioscoreae Rhizoma 80 g, Poria 60 g, Alismatis Rhizoma 60 g. Procedure: pulverize the above six ingredients to fine powder, sift and mix well. To each 100 g of the powder add 35 – 50 g of refined honey and a quantity of water to make water – honeyed pills and dry; or add 80 – 110 g of refined honey to make small or big honeyed pills. Action: To replenish yin of the kidney. Indications: deficiency of the kidney marked by dizziness, tinnitus, aching and limpness of the loins and knees, consumptive fever, night sweating, seminal emission or diabetes.

Rehmanniae Radix Preparata is the preparata of the fresh or dried tuberous root of *Rehmannia glutinosa* Libosch. (Fam. Scrophulariaceae). It mainly contains iridoid compounds, e. g. catalpol. Corni Fructus (processed with wine) is the dried and mature flesh of *Cornus officinalis* Sieb. et Zucc. (Fam. Cornaceae). It contains loganin, ursolic acid, etc. Moutan

Cortex is the dried root bark of *Paeonia suffruticosa* Andr. (Fam. Ranunculaceae). It mainly contains paeonol, paeoniflorin, volatile oil, etc. Dioscoreae Rhizoma is the dried rhizome of *Dioscorea opposita* Thunb. (Fam. Dioscoreaceae). It mainly contains starch, phlegm, e. g. mannan, phytic acid. Poria is the dried sclertium of *Poria cocos* (Schw.) Wolf (Fam. Polyporaceae). It mainly contains β – pachyman, pachymic acid, ebricoic acid, tumulosic acid, pinicolic acid, etc. Alismatis Rhizoma is the dried tuber of *Alisma orientalis* (Sam.) Juzep. (Fam. Alismataceae). It mainly contains tetracyclic triterpenoids, e. g. alisol A, B, C.

The principal drug Rehmanniae Radix Preparata has the effect of mourishing kidney yin and producing essence. Fructus Corni (processed with wine) and Dioscoreae Rhizoma are two minister drugs which the former serves to nourish blood, liver and kidney yin as well as to astringe the essence, the later is used to invigorate vital energy and spleen yin, and to preserve the essence with its astringent nature. The above three aim at invigorating kidney, liver and spleen yin respectively. Moutan Cortex serves to purge liver fire by clearing away heat evil and cooling blood. Poria is used to eliminate spleen dampness evil, help Dioscoreae Rhizoma to invigorate vital energy and spleen. Alismatis Rhizoma serves to purge kidney fire by eliminating dampness evil, and to minimize the greasy nature of Rehmanniae Radix Preparata. The above three drugs are assistant and guide in the prescription. This prescription is characterized by nourishing three yin with three drugs and purging asthenia fire evil with another three drugs. The quality analysis should be carried out under the guidance of the theory of TCM.

2. In microscopical identification, use glycerin – acetic acid TS as mountant to observe starch granules and irregular branched. Other characters can be observed by adding dropwise a adequate quantity of dilute glycerin after the disposal of chloral hydrate TS. Under the microscope, starch granules in Dioscoreae Rhizoma triangular – ovoid or oblong, 24 – 40 μm in diameter, hilum short cleft or V – shaped; raphides of calcium oxalate thick and long, exist in mucous cells. Irregular branched masses in Poria colourless, dissolved in chloral hydrate solution; hyphae colourless, 4 – 6 μm in diameter. Parenchyma of Rehmanniae Radix Preparata grayish – brown to black – brown, cells mostly shrunken, and each containing a brown nucleus – like mass. Clusters of calcium oxalate in Moutan Cortex occurring in colourless parenchymatous cells, sometimes several clusters arranged in rows. Epidermal cells of pericarp in Corni Fructus (processed with wine) orange – yellow, polygonal in surface view, with somewhat beaded anticlinal walls. Parenchymatous cells of Alismatis Rhizoma subrounded, with elliptical pits, gathered into pit groups. Endodermis cells is thicker and lignificated, with somewhat beaded anticlinal walls and few and scattered thin elliptical pits. (Figure 6 – 2)

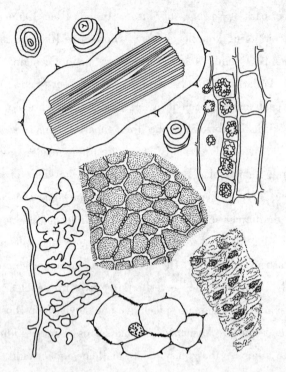

Figure 6 – 2　Microscopical Identification of Liuwei Dihuang Pills

. Rehmanniae Radix Preparata parenchymatous cells　2. Corni Fructus（processed with wine）carp epidermis cells

3. Moutan Cortex calcium oxalate cluster crystal　4. Moutan Cortex cork cells

5. Dioscoreae Rhizoma calcium oxalate acicular crystal　6. Dioscoreae Rhizoma starch grains

7. Poria irregular branched masses　8. Alismatis Rhizoma parenchymatous cells

3. The chemical structure of loganin and paeonol

loganin　　　　　　　　　　paeonol

4. The preparation of reagents

（1）Glycerin Dilute TS　Dilute 33 ml of glycerin with water to 100 ml. Add a small piece of camphor or a drop of liquefied phenol.

（2）Chloral Hydrate TS　Dissolve 50 g of chloral hydrate in a mixture of 15 ml of water and 10 ml of glycerin.

（3）Glycerin – acetic Acid TS　Mix 1 volume of glycerin, 1 volume of 50% acetic acid and 1 volume of water.

实验十八　牛黄解毒片的理化鉴别及羟基蒽醌的含量测定

【目的要求】

1. 掌握中药理化鉴别的常用方法。

2. 掌握采用分光光度法测定羟基蒽醌的原理及方法。

【原理】

利用理化方法及薄层色谱法鉴别中药制剂的处方。利用羟基蒽醌衍生物在碱性溶液中生成红色或紫红色物质在500～530nm有最大吸收，采用分光光度法，以大黄素为对照品，测定羟基蒽醌的含量。

【仪器、试剂与药品】

1. **仪器**　分光光度计、超声波清洗器、恒温水浴锅。

2. **材料**　硅胶H薄层板（5cm×10cm）、硅胶G薄层板（5cm×10cm）、立式展开槽（10cm×10cm）、量瓶（25ml）、锥形瓶（50ml）、刻度移液管（5ml、1ml）、分液漏斗、漏斗、蒸发皿、滴管、试管、乳钵、刀片。

3. **试剂**　95%乙醇、甲醇、正己烷、三氯甲烷、乙醚、石油醚（30～60℃）、甲酸乙酯、乙酸乙酯、甲酸、醋酸、5%氢氧化钠、30%过氧化氢、10%草酸铵、稀盐酸、10%醋酸、饱和氯化钡试液、5%氢氧化钠-2%氢氧化铵（1∶1）混合碱液。

4. **药品**　大黄素对照品甲醇溶液（1mg/ml、0.1mg/ml）、胆酸对照品乙醇溶液（1mg/ml）；大黄对照药材；牛黄解毒片（市售品）。

【实验内容】

1. 大黄的鉴别

（1）取本品10片，刮去糖衣，研细，取样品粉末1.0g，置锥形瓶中，加乙醇15ml，温热20分钟，滤过。取滤液2ml，加5%氢氧化钠试液，即显橙红色，再加30%过氧化氢溶液，加热红色不褪，加酸成酸性时，则红色消褪，变为黄色。

（2）取本品1片，研细，加甲醇20ml，超声处理15分钟，滤过，取滤液10ml，蒸干，残渣加水10ml使溶解，加盐酸1ml，加热回流30分钟，放冷，用乙醚振摇提取2次，每次20ml，合并乙醚液，蒸干，残渣加三氯甲烷2ml使溶解，作为供试品溶液。另取大黄对照药材0.1g，同法制作对照药材溶液。再取大黄素对照品，加甲醇制成每1ml含1mg的溶液，作为对照品溶液。吸取上述三种溶液各4μl，分别点于同一以羧甲基纤维素钠为黏合剂的硅胶H薄层板上，以石油醚（30～60℃）-甲酸乙酯-甲酸（15∶5∶1）的上层溶液为展开剂，展开，取出，晾干，置紫外光灯（365nm）下检视。供试品色谱中，在与和对照药材色谱相应的位置上，显相同的5个橙黄色荧光斑点；在与对照品色谱相应的位置上，显相同的橙黄色荧光斑点；置氨蒸气中薰后，日光下检视，斑点变为红色。

2. 人工牛黄的鉴别　取本品2片，研细，加三氯甲烷10ml研磨，滤过。滤液蒸干，残渣加乙醇0.5ml使溶解，作为供试品溶液。另取胆酸对照品，加乙醇制成每1ml

含 1mg 的溶液，作为对照品溶液。吸取上述两种溶液各 5 μl，分别点于同一硅胶 G 薄层板上，以正己烷－乙酸乙酯－甲醇－醋酸（20：25：3：2）的上层溶液为展开剂，展开，取出，晾干，喷以 10% 硫酸乙醇溶液，在 105℃ 加热约 10 分钟，置紫外光灯（365nm）下检视。供试品色谱中，在与对照品色谱相应的位置上，显相同颜色的荧光斑点。

3. 冰片的鉴别 取本品 1 片，研细，进行微量升华，所得的白色升华物，加新配制的 1% 香草醛硫酸溶液 1~2 滴，液滴边缘渐显玫瑰红色。

4. 石膏的鉴别 取样品粉末 1.0g，置锥形瓶中，加入稀盐酸 15ml，加热 5 分钟，滤过。取滤液 2ml，加草酸铵试液即发生沉淀，沉淀应不溶于醋酸，但可溶于盐酸中。另取滤液 2ml，加氯化钡试液，即发生白色沉淀。沉淀应不溶于盐酸中。

$$Ca^{2+}+(COO)^{2-} \longrightarrow Ca^{2+}(COO)_2 \downarrow \xrightarrow{H^+} Ca^{2+}+(COOH)_2$$

$$SO_4^{2-}+Ba^{2+} \longrightarrow BaSO_4 \downarrow$$

5. 羟基蒽醌的含量测定

（1）标准曲线的制备 分别吸取大黄素对照品甲醇溶液（0.1mg/ml）0.5，1.0，2.0，3.0，4.0ml 于 25ml 量瓶中，加 5% 氢氧化钠－2% 氢氧化铵混合碱液至刻度，摇匀，在水浴上加热 5 分钟，放置 10 分钟至室温，以混合碱液为空白，在 530nm 处测定吸收度，绘出浓度－吸收度曲线，并计算回归方程及相关系数。

（2）供试品溶液的绘制 精密称取样品粉末 0.5g，置 50ml 锥形瓶中，加入三氯甲烷 25ml，超声提取 3 次，每次 5 分钟，滤过，滤渣再加三氯甲烷 15ml，超声提取 5 分钟，滤过，合并两次提取液，于分液漏斗中，分别用 5% NaOH－2% NH₄OH 混合碱液 15ml、5ml 振摇提取两次，直至混合碱液无色，合并混合碱液，弃去三氯甲烷液，将混合碱液在水浴上加热 5 分钟至三氯甲烷挥散尽，放置 10 分钟，移入 25ml 量瓶中，加 5% 氢氧化钠－2% 氢氧化铵混合碱液至刻度，摇匀，作为供试品溶液。

（3）样品测定 以 5% NaOH－2% NH₄OH 混合碱液为空白，将供试品溶液与大黄素对照品甲醇溶液（0.1mg/ml）在 530nm 处同时测定吸收度。按外标一点法，计算如下：

样品中相当于大黄素的游离羟基蒽醌量 ＝

$$对照品溶液每~ml~含有大黄素的量 \times \frac{供试品溶液吸收度 \times 25ml}{对照品溶液吸收液 \times 样品称取量} \times 100\%$$

【实验记录】

1. 记录牛黄解毒片的鉴别实验结果，绘制薄层色谱图并算出主要斑点的 R_f 值。

2. 记录含量测定实验数据，计算羟基蒽醌的含量。

【思考题】

1. 简述采用分光光度法测定羟基蒽醌的原理。

2. 能否采用分光光度法测定牛黄解毒片中结合型羟基蒽醌含量？试设计测定方案。

【相关资料】

1. 牛黄解毒片的处方：牛黄 5g，大黄 200g，黄芩 150g，石膏 200g，雄黄 50g，冰片 28g，桔梗 100g，甘草 50g。制法：以上八味，雄黄水飞成细粉；大黄粉碎成细粉；人工牛黄、冰片研细；其余黄芩等四味加水煎煮两次，每次 2 小时，合并煎液，滤过，滤液浓缩成稠膏，加入大黄、雄黄粉末，制粒，干燥，再加入人工牛黄、冰片粉末，混匀，压制成 1000 片（大片）或 1500 片（小片），或包糖衣或薄膜衣，即得。功能与主治：清热解毒。用于火热内盛，咽喉肿痛，牙龈肿痛，口舌生疮，目赤肿痛。

2. 胆酸（cholic acid）和去氧胆酸（deoxycholic acid）均是人工牛黄中主要有效成分，具有解痉、降压、镇痛等多种药理活性，它们在药理作用方面有协同作用。

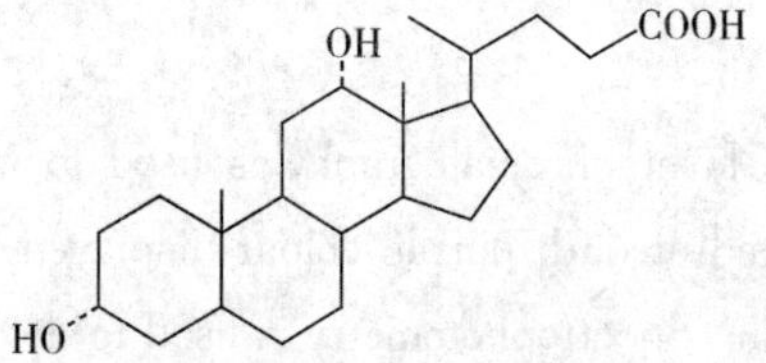

去氧胆酸胆酸 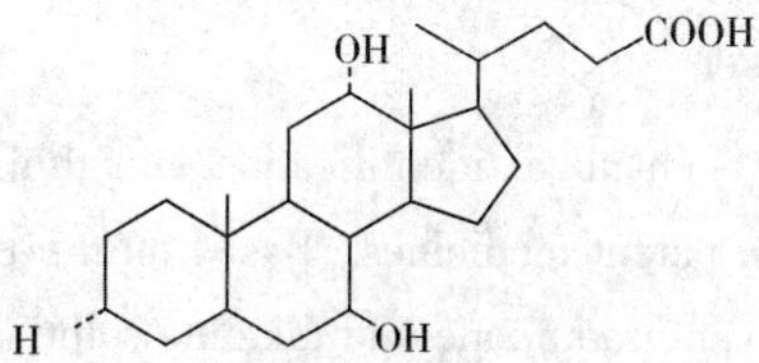　　　　　　　　　　　　　胆酸

3. 大黄的主要成分为蒽醌类衍生物，少部分以游离态蒽醌衍生物存在，如大黄酸、大黄素、大黄酚、大黄素甲醚、芦荟大黄素等，大部分以结合蒽醌衍生物的形式存在。结合蒽醌衍生物为游离蒽醌的糖苷，或双蒽酮苷。结合蒽醌的糖的部分具有保护作用，可通过消化道，抵达大肠，再经酶的作用分解成苷元，刺激大肠，增加肠的蠕动，是大黄的主要泻下成分，其中以双蒽酮苷的泻下作用最强，主要有番泻苷 A、B、C、D 等。而游离蒽醌衍生物则不具有泻下作用，仅显示强的抗菌作用。评价大黄及其制剂的质量须从这两类成分来考虑。

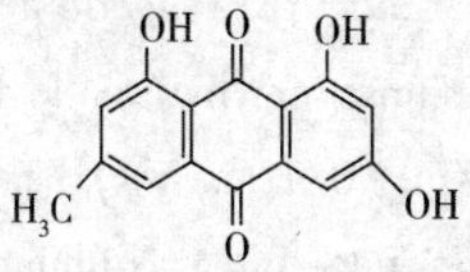

大黄素（emodin） 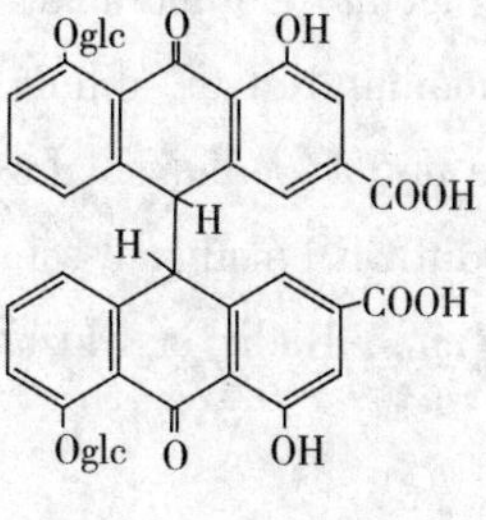　　　　　　　　　　番泻苷 A（sennoside A）

4. Auterhoff 发现，将羟基蒽醌用含有 2% 氨水的氢氧化钠的混合碱液处理，得到下式而显色，λ_{max} 在 510~530 nm 之间，并且在酸性条件下不褪色。因此，采用 5% 氢氧化钠－2% 氢氧化铵混合碱液作为显色剂。

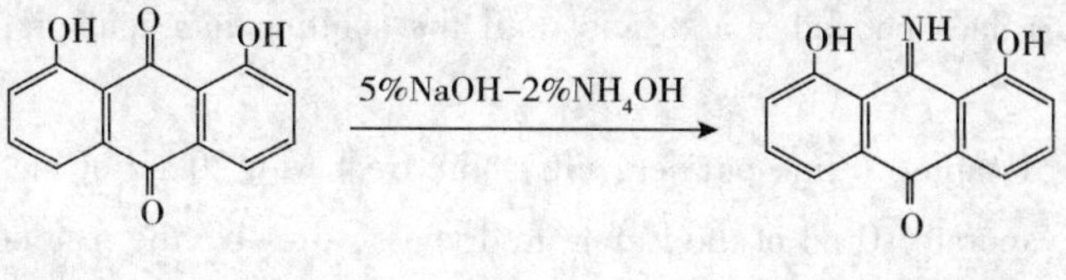

5%NaOH－2%NH₄OH

Experiment 18   Physical – chemical Identification of Niuhuang

Jiedu Tablets and Determination of Hydroxyanthraquinone

Purpose

1. To grasp the method of identification of the physical – chemical properties of Traditional Chinese medicine.

2. To master the principle and method of spectrophotometry in the assay ofhydroxyanthraquinone.

Principle

The physical – chemical identification and thin layer chromatography is used to identify traditional Chinese patent medicines. Based on the red or dark purple colour displayed by the reaction of hydroxyanthraquinone and alkaline solution. Spectrophotometry is used to determine hydroxyanthraquinone at 500 – 530 nm, which was the maximum absorbant wavelength of emodin CRS developed by alkaline solution.

Apparatus, materials, reagents and drugs

1. Apparatus: spectrophotometer, ultrasonic surge, water bath.

2. Materials: Silica gel H – TLC plate (5 cm × 10 cm), Silica gel G – TLC plate (5 cm × 10 cm), vertical developing chamber (10 cm × 10 cm), volumetric flask (25 ml), conical flask (50 ml), transfer pipette (5 ml, 1 ml), separating funnel, funnel, evaporating – dish, dropper, test tube, mortar, blade.

3. Reagents: 95% ethanol, methanol, n – hexane, chloroform, ether, petroleum ether (30 ~ 60 ℃), ethyl acetate, formic acid, acetic acid, 5% sodium hydroxide, 30% hydrogen peroxide, 10% ammonium oxalate, dilute hydrochloric acid, 10% acetic acid, saturated barium chloride, mixture of 5% sodium hydroxide – 2% ammonium hydroxide (1 : 1).

4. Drugs: emodin CRS methanol solution (1 mg/ml, 0.1 mg/ml), cholic acid CRS ethanol solution (1 mg/ml); Radix et Rhizoma Rhei reference drug; Niuhuang Jiedu Pian (for sale).

Procedure

1. Identification of Rhei Radix et Rhizoma

(1) To 10 tablets, removed the sugar coats and grind finely. Dissolve 1.0 g of the power in 15 ml ethanol to conical flask, heat warmly for 20 minutes and filter. Measure 2 ml of the filtrate, add 5% sodium hydroxide, a orange – yellow is produced, add 30% hydrogen peroxide, heat, the color does not fade, add acid until the solution has acid property, the colour fade, turn yellow.

(2) Pulverize 1 tablet to fine powder, ultrasonic treat with 20 ml of methanol for 15 minutes and filter. Evaporate 10 ml of the filtrate to dryness, dissolve the residue in 10 ml of wa-

ter, add 1 ml of hydrochloric acid, heat under reflux for 30 minutes, allow to cool, extract with two 20 ml quantities of ether. Combine the ether extracts, evaporate to dryness, and dissolve the residue in 2 ml of chloroform as the test solution. Prepare a reference drug solution in the same manner using 0. 1 g of Rhei Radix et Rhizoma reference drug. Using silica gel H mixed with sodium carboxymethylcellulose solution as the coating substance, and the upper layer of petroleum ether (30 ~ 60 ℃), ethyl formate and formic acid (15 : 5 : 1) as the mobile phase. Apply separately to the plate 4 μl of each of the above two solutions and emodin CRS methanol solution (1 mg/ml) . After developing and removal of the plate, dry it in air, examine under ultraviolet light at 365 nm. The five orange yellow fluorescent spots in the chromatogram obtain with the test solution correspond in position and colour to the spots in the chromatogram obtained with the reference drug solution. The orange yellow fluorescent spot in the chromatogram obtained with test solution corresponds in position and colour to the spot in the chromatogram obtained with the reference solution. The spots turn red in daylight on exposure to ammonia vapour.

2. Identification of Bovis Calculus Artifactus

Pulverize 2 tablets to fine powder with 10 ml of chloroform and filter. Evaporate the filtrate to dry, dissolve the residue in 0. 5 ml of ethanol as the test solution. Apply separately to the plate 5 μl of each of the test solution and cholic acid CRS ethanol solution, using the upper layer of n – hexane, ethyl acetate, methanol and acetic acid (20 : 25 : 3 : 2) as the mobile phase. After developing and removal of the plate, dry it in air, spray with 10% solution of sulfuric acid in ethanol, heat at 105 ℃ for about 10 minutes and examine under ultraviolet at 365 nm. The fluorescent spot in the chromatogram obtained with the test solution corresponds in position and colour to the spot in the chromatogram obtained with the reference solution.

3. Identification of Borneolum

Triturate 1 tablet to fine powder and carry outmicrosublimation. To the white sublimate obtained add 1 – 2 drops of freshly prepared 1% vanillin solution in sulfuric acid, a rose – red colour is produced gradually on the edge of liquid drop.

4. Identification of Gypsum Fibrosum

Dissolve 1. 0 g of the powder in 15 ml dilute hydrochloric acid to conical flask, heat for 5 minutes, filter. Add ammonium oxalate to 2 ml of the filtrate, precipitation is produced. The precipitation should not dissolve in acetic acid but can dissolve in hydrochloric acid. Add barium chloride solution to 2 ml of the filtrate, white precipitation is produced. The precipitation does not dissolve in hydrochloric acid.

$$Ca^{2+}+(COO)^{2-} \longrightarrow Ca(COO)_2 \downarrow \xrightarrow{H^+} Ca^{2+}+(COOH)_2$$

$$SO4^{2-}+Ba^{2+} \longrightarrow BaSO_4 \downarrow$$

5. Assay ofhydroxyanthraquinone

Preparation of standard curve　Transfer accurately 0. 5, 1. 0, 2. 0, 3. 0, 4. 0 ml emodin CRS methanol solution (0. 1 mg/ml) into 25 ml volumetric flasks separately, dilute with 5% sodium – hydroxide – 2% ammonium – hydroxide to volume, mix well, put on water bath for 5 minutes, allow to stand for ten minutes and cool to room temperature, use the mixed base solution as the blank, measure the absorbance at 530 nm, plot the curve of absorbance to concentration, calculate the regression equation and correlation coefficient.

Preparation of test solution　Weigh accurately 0. 5 g of the powder to conical flask, add 25 ml of chloroform, ultrasonic treat for 3 times, each time for 5 minutes, filter. Resolve the residue with 15 ml chloroform, ultrasonic treat for 5 minutes, filter, combine the filtrates to separating funnel, extract with 15 ml, 5 ml mixture of 5% sodium – hydroxide – 2% ammonium – oxalate separately, shake thoroughly until the mixture is colorless, combine the mixture, discard the chloroform, put the mixture on water bath to evaporate the chloroform, allow to stand for ten minutes, transfer the mixture to a 25 ml volumetric flask, dilute with mixture of 5% sodium hydroxide – 2% ammonium hydroxide to volume and shake well for use.

Determination of sample　Use 5% sodium hydroxide – 2% ammonium hydroxide as the blank, measure the absorbance of the test solution and the reference solution at 530 nm, calculate the content according to external standard of one point as follow:

Freehydroxyanthraquinone in sample which is equal to emodin =

$$\frac{\text{the content of emodin in reference solution per ml} \times \text{the absorbance of test solution} \times 25\text{ml} \times 100\%}{\text{the absorbance of reference solution} \times \text{the weight of sample}}$$

Experiment records

1. Record the identification test, plot the TLC chromatograms and calculate the R_f value of major spots.

2. Record the assay data and calculate the content of freehydroxyanthraquinone.

Questions

1. Describe the principle of determininghydroxyanthraquinone by spectrophotometry.

2. Could we determine the combinedhydroxyanthraquinone in Niuhuang Jiedu Tablets by spectrophotometry? And try to design the experimental scheme of determination.

Related materials

1. Ingredients of Niuhuang Jiedu Tablets: Bovis Calculus Artifactus 5 g, Realgar 50 g, Gypsum Fibrosunm 200 g, Rhei Radix et Rhizoma 200 g, Scutellariae Radix 150 g, Platycodi Radix 100 g, Borneolum Syntheticum 25 g, Glycyrrhizae Radix et Rhizoma 50 g. Procedure: Levigate Realgar to very fine powder, pulverize Rhei Radix et Rhizoma to fine power and triturate Bovis Calculus Artifactus and Borneolum Syntheticum to fine powder. Decoct the other four ingredients with water twice, two hours for each. Combine the decoctions and filter. Evaporate the filtrate to a thick extract, add the powder of Rhei Radix et Rhizoma and Realgar, make granules and dry. Add the powders of Bovis Calculus Artifactus Borneolum Syntheticum, mix

well, make to 1000 tablets (big tablets) or 1500 tablets (small tablets); or coat the tablets with sugar or film. Action: To clear heat and remove toxin. Indication: patterns of internally exuberant wind – fire – heat, manifested as swollen sore throat, swollen painful gums, mouth and tongue sores, red painful swelling eyes.

2. Cholic acid and deoxycholic acid are the main active constituents of Bovis Calculus Artifactus, they exhibit synergic effect in pharmacological effects such as anticonvulsion, antihypertention, ect.

3. The main components of Rhei Radix et Rhizoma are hydroxyanthraquinones, including free hydroxyanthraquinones and combined hydroxyanthraquinones. The free hydroxyanthraquinones such as rhein, emodin, chrysophanol, aloe – emodin, and physcion, have the antimicrobial activities, but no lapactic effect. The lapactic effect of Rhei Radix et Rhizoma is due to the combined hydroxyanthraquinones such as sennoside A, B, C, D etc. The quality evaluation of Rhei Radix et Rhizoma Rhei and its preparations depends on these two kinds of hydroxyanthraquinones.

4. Auterhoff detected that hydroxyanthraquinone being disposed with the mixture solution of 2% ammonia solution and 5% sodium hydroxide disply certain colour and come to the following formula. λ_{max} is at 510 – 530 nm and the colour does not fade in the acid condition. So we usually use 2% ammonium – hydroxide as colour – developing reagent.

第七章　设计性实验

Chapter 7　Design Experiment

实验十九　设计复方丹参片和滴丸的质量分析方法

【目的要求】

1. 掌握常用分析方法在中药制剂鉴别与含量测定中的应用。

2. 设计本品的定性鉴别和含量测定分析方案。

【处方】

丹参450g，三七141g，冰片8g。

【制法】

以上三味，丹参加乙醇加热回流1.5小时，提取液滤过，滤液回收乙醇并浓缩至适量，备用；药渣加50%乙醇加热回流1.5小时，提取液滤过，滤液回收乙醇并浓缩至适量，备用；药渣加水煎煮2小时，煎液滤过，滤液浓缩至适量。三七粉碎成细粉，与上述浓缩液和适量的辅料制成颗粒，干燥。冰片研细，与上述颗粒混匀，压制成

1000 片。包糖衣或薄膜衣，即得。

【性状】

本品为糖衣片或薄膜衣片，除去包衣后显棕色至棕褐色，气芳香，味微苦。

【功能与主治】

活血化瘀，理气止痛。用于气滞血瘀所致的胸痹，症见胸闷、心前区刺痛；冠心病心绞痛见上述证候者。

【质量分析方法设计要求】

1. 熟悉本品的处方、制法以及性状。

2. 参考相关文献和所学知识，设计处方中药味的鉴别实验方法，主要包括鉴别依据、鉴别方法、反应原理、实验条件、供试品溶液和对照品溶液的制备方法、实验操作过程、预期结果等。要写明所用对照品或对照药材，以及鉴别方法。

3. 设计处方中主药有效成分或指标性成分的含量测定方案，主要包括测定依据、测定方法、测定原理、实验条件、供试品溶液和对照品溶液的制备方法、实验操作过程，含量计算，预期结果等。写明样品提取净化方法、所测成分、测定条件。试进行方法学考察实验的设计。

Experiment 19   Design the Analysis Experiment
for Compound Salvia Tablets and Drop Pill

Purpose

1. To master the commonly analytical methods in the identification and determination of the content of traditional Chinese patent medicine.

2. To design the experiments of qualitative identification and assay for the patent medicine.

Ingredients

Salviae Miltiorrhizae Radix et Rhizama 450 g, Notoginseng Radix et Rhizama 141 g, Borneolum Syntheticum 8 g.

Procedure

Heat under reflux Salviae Miltiorrhizae Radix et Rhizama with ethanol for 1. 5 hours, filter the extract, recover ethanol and concentrate the filtrate to a quantity for use; heat under reflux the residue with 50% ethanol for 1. 5 hours, filter the extract, recover ethanol and concentrate the filtrate to a quantity for use; decoct the residue with water for 2 hours, filter the decoction, concentrate the filtrate to a quantity. Pulverize Notoginseng Radix et Rhizama to fine powder, mix with the above concentrate and a quantity of subsidiary stuffs to make granules and dry. Grind Borneolum Syntheticum to fine powder, mix well with the above granules to make 1000 tablets. Coat with sugar or film.

Description

Sugar or film coated tablets, with brown to sepia core; odour, aromatic; taste, slightly bitter.

Action and Indications

Action: To activate blood, resolve stasis, regulate qi and relieve pain.

Indications: Chest bi disorder due to qi stagnation and blood stasis, manifested as oppression in the chest, stabbing pain in the precordium; Angina pectoris in coronary heart disease with the symptoms described above.

Indications: thoracic obstruction caused by qi – stagnancy and blood stasis, manifested as sensation of stuffiness in the chest, precordial stabbing pain, angina pectoris of coronary heart disease marked by above symptoms.

Design Requirements of the Qualitative Analysis

1. To be familiar with ingredients, procedureand description of this tablet.

2. To refer to the correlated literaturess and knowledge that we have learned, design the identification experiment of each ingredient, mainly including identification basis, identification method, reaction principle, experimental condition, preparation methods of the test solution and the reference solution, operation, and expected result etc. To give clear indication of the CRS or the reference drug and identification methods used in the experiment.

3. To design the assay experiments of the effective components or characteristic components of major drugs in ingredients, mainly including determination basis, determination method, determination principle, experimental condition, preparation methods of the test solution and the reference solution, operation, calculation and expected result etc. To give clear indication of extraction and purification methods of the sample, measured components, and determination condition. Try to design the experiment for investigation of methodology.

实验二十 设计消渴丸的质量分析方法

【目的要求】

1. 掌握常用分析方法在中成药鉴别与含量测定中的应用。

2. 设计本品的定性鉴别、检查和含量测定分析方案。

【处方】

葛根，地黄，黄芪，天花粉，玉米须，山药，南五味子，格列本脲。

【制法】

以上八味，葛根、地黄、天花粉、玉米须加水煎煮5小时，滤过，滤液浓缩至适量；黄芪、山药、南五味子粉碎成细粉，与上述部分浓缩液拌匀，干燥，粉碎，过筛，混匀，用剩余的浓缩液制丸，干燥，加入格列本脲，用黑氧化铁和滑石粉的糊精液包衣，制成1000丸，即得。

【性状】

本品为黑色的包衣浓缩水丸；味甘、酸、微涩。

【功能与主治】

滋肾养阴，益气生津。用于气阴两虚所致的消渴病，症见多饮、多尿、多食、消瘦、体倦乏力、睡眠差、腰痛；2 型糖尿病见上述证候者。

【质量分析方法设计要求】

1. 熟悉本品的处方、制法以及性状。

2. 参考相关文献和所学知识，设计处方中药味的鉴别实验方法，主要包括鉴别依据，鉴别方法、反应原理、实验条件、供试品溶液和对照溶液的制备方法、实验操作过程和预期结果等。要写明所用对照品或对照药材鉴别方法。

3. 设计本品的检查项目及方案。

4. 设计处方中主药有效成分或指标性成分的含量测定方案，主要包括测定依据、测定方法、测定原理、实验条件、供试品溶液和对照品溶液的制备方法、实验操作过程、含量计算和预期结果等。写明样品提取净化方法、所测成分、测定条件。试进行方法学考察实验的设计。

Experiment 20　Design of Analysis Experiment for Xiaokewan Pills

Purpose

1. To master the commonly used analytical methods in identification and assay of traditional Chinese patent medicine.

2. Design the experiments of qualitative identification, test and assay for the patent medicine.

Ingredients

Puerariae Lobatae Radix, Rehmanniae Radix, Astragali Mongolici Radix, Trichosanthis Radix, Zeae Maydis Stylus, Dioscoreae Oppositae Rhizoma , Schisandrae Sphenanthrae Fructus, Glibenclamide.

Procedure

Decoct Puerariae Lobatae Radix, Rehmanniae Radix, Trichosanthis Radix and Maydis Stigma with water for five hours, combine the decoctions, and filter. Concentrate the filtrate to the amount. Pulverize Astragali Mongolici Radix, Dioscoreae Oppositae Rhizoma and Kadsura Japonica L. to fine powder. Mix the fine power with the above decoctions thoroughly, dry, pulverize, sift, mix thoroughly. Make pills with surplus decoctions, dry and add a quantity of glibenclamide, coat with ferric oxide black and pulvis talci in cycloamylose solution, make into 1000 pills.

Description

Black coating concentrated water pills; taste, sweet, sour, slightly astringent.

Action and Indications

Actions: To nourish kidney, yin and qi, and engender fluid.

Indications: Wasting – thirst due to dual deficiency of qi and yin, manifested as increased water intake, increased urination. increased food intake, weight loss, fatigue, lack of strength, restless sleep, and lower back pain; Type II diabetes with the symptoms described above.

Requirments of Experiment Design

1. To be familiar with ingredients, procedure and description of this pill.

2. To refer to the correlated literaturess and knowledge that we have learned, design the identification experiment of each ingredient, mainly including identification basis, identification method, reaction principle, experimental condition, preparation methods of the test solution and the reference solution, operation, and expected result etc。 To give clear indication of the CRS or the reference drug and identification methods used in the experiment.

3. According to the test requirment of foreign matter for Mixture, design the test item for the mixture.

4. To design the assay experiments of the effective components or characteristic components of major drugs in ingredients, mainly including determination basis, determination method, determination principle, experimental condition, preparation methods of the test solution and the reference solution, operation, calculation and expected result etc. To give clear indication of extraction and purification methods of the sample, measured components, and determination condition. Try to design the experiment for investigation of methodology.

附　录

常用薄层色谱显色剂的配制和使用

一、通用显色剂

1. **碘蒸气**　将薄层板放入底部有少许晶体碘片的密闭容器，许多化合物产生棕色斑点。

2. **硫酸试液**　常用5%、10%硫酸乙醇溶液。喷10%浓硫酸的乙醇溶液，105℃烘烤至斑点清晰。

3. **碘化钾–碘**　取碘0.5g与碘化钾1.5g，加水25ml使溶解，即得，喷雾后许多化合物显棕黄色。

4. **磷钼酸试剂**　取磷钼酸5g，加无水乙醇使溶解成100ml，即得。喷后于105℃烘烤，还原性物质显蓝色斑点。

5. **铁氰化钾**　取铁氰化钾1g，加水10ml使溶解，即得。本液应临时新配。

二、生物碱及含氮化合物

1. **碘化铋钾试液**　取次硝酸铋0.85g，加冰醋酸10ml与水40ml溶解后，加碘化钾溶液（4→10）20ml，摇匀，即得。

2. **改良碘化铋钾**　取碘化铋钾试液1ml，加0.6mol/L盐酸溶液2ml，加水至10ml，即得。

3. **碘化汞钾试液**　取二氯化汞1.36g，加水60ml使溶解，另取碘化钾5g，加水10ml使溶解，将两液混合，加水稀释至100ml，即得。

4. **碘化钾试液**　取碘化钾16.5g，加水使溶解成100ml，即得。本液应临时新配。

5. **稀碘化铋钾试液**　取次硝酸铋0.85g，加冰醋酸10ml与水40ml溶解后，即得。临用前取5ml，加碘化钾溶液（4→10）5ml，再加冰醋酸20ml，加水稀释至100ml，即得。

6. **对–二甲氨基苯甲醛试液**　取对–二甲氨基苯甲醛0.125g，加无氮硫酸65ml与水35ml的冷混合液溶解后，加三氯化铁试液0.05ml，摇匀，即得。本液配制后7日即不适用。

三、糖类

1. **苯胺–邻苯二甲酸**　取0.93g苯胺和1.66g邻苯二甲酸，加100ml水饱和的正丁醇，即得。不同种类的糖会出现不同颜色的斑点，对还原糖的检出灵敏度高。

2. **α-萘酚试液** 取15%的α-萘酚乙醇溶液10.5ml，缓慢加硫酸6.5ml，混匀后再加乙醇40.5ml及水4ml，混匀，即得。

3. **茴香醛试液** 取茴香醛0.5ml，加入醋酸50ml使溶解，加硫酸1ml，摇匀，即得。本液应临用新制。喷后100~105℃加热，不同种类糖显不同颜色。

四、酚类化合物

1. **重氮苯磺酸试液** 取对氨基苯磺酸1.57g，加水80ml与稀盐酸10ml，在水浴上加热溶解后，放冷至15℃，缓慢加入亚硝酸钠溶液（1→10）6.5ml，随加随搅拌，再加水稀释至100ml，即得。本液应临用新制。酚类化合物呈现红色斑点。

2. **间苯三酚-盐酸试液** 取间苯三酚0.1g，加乙醇1ml，再加盐酸9ml，混匀。本液应临用新制。

3. **三氯化铁试剂** 取三氯化铁9g，加水使溶解成100ml，即得。酚类呈蓝色或绿色。

4. **三氯化铝试剂** 取三氯化铝9g，加乙醇使溶解成100ml，即得。用于检测黄铜。

五、醌类化合物

醋酸镁试剂 取醋酸镁0.5g，加甲醇使溶解成100ml，即得。90℃加热5分钟醌类化合物即可显色。

六、萜类化合物

香草醛-硫酸试液 取香草醛0.1g，加硫酸10ml使溶解，即得。喷后加热至显色。

七、挥发油

1. **香草醛-硫酸试液** 取香草醛0.1g，加硫酸10ml使溶解，即得。喷后加热至显色。

2. **茴香醛-浓硫酸试液** 取茴香醛0.5ml，加入醋酸50ml使溶解，加硫酸1ml，摇匀，即得。本液应临用新制。喷后100~105℃加热。

八、甾体化合物

醋酐-浓硫酸 取5ml醋酐和5ml浓硫酸，在冷却条件下，混合后加入无水乙醇至50ml，即得。本液应临用新制。喷后100℃加热10分钟，用于检测甾醇、三萜皂苷类。

九、氨基酸

茚三酮试液 取茚三酮2g，加乙醇使溶解成100ml，即得。

十、有机酸类

1. 溴酚蓝试剂 取溴酚蓝 0.1g，加 0.05mol/L 氢氧化钠溶液 3.0ml 使溶解，再加水稀释至 200ml，即得。

2. 溴甲酚绿（蓝）指示剂 取溴甲酚蓝 0.04g，加乙醇使溶解成 100ml，加 0.1mol/L 氢氧化钠溶液至蓝色刚出现。

Appendix   The preparation and usage of commonly used TLC colorant

1. General colorant

（1）Iodine vapour   Putting thin layer plate in basal part of closed container where some crystal iodine are there, many chemical compounds appear brown spot.

（2）Sulphuric acid TS   Frequently used 5%, 10% sulphuric acid – ethanol solution. To puff 10% concentrated sulfuric acid ethanol solution, bake to the spot clear at 105 ℃.

（3）Iodine potassium – iodine TS   Dissolve 0.5 g of iodine and 1.5 g of potassium iodine in 25 ml of water.

（4）Phosphomdybdic acid TS   Dissolve 5 g phosphomdybdic acid in ethanol to make 100 ml. After puff bake to the spot clear at 105 ℃. Reducing substances appear blue spot.

（5）Potassium ferricyanide TS   Dissolve 1 g of potassium ferricyanide in water to 100 ml. This solution should be freshly prepared.

2. Colorant for alkaloid and nitrogenous compound

（1）Potassium iodobismuthate TS   Dissolve 0.85 g of bismuth subnitrate in a mixture of 10 ml of glacial acetic acid and 40 ml of water, and then add 20 ml of potassium iodide solution （4→10）and mix well.

（2）Potassium iodobismuthate modified TS   Dissolve 1 ml of bismuth subnitrate in 2 ml of 0.6 mol/L hydrochloric acid and in water to make 10 ml.

（3）Mercuric potassium iodide TS   Dissolve 1.36 g of hydrargyri bichloridum, in 60 ml of water, and dissolve 5 g of potassium iodide in 10 ml of water. Mix these solutions and dilute with water to 100 ml.

（4）Potassium iodide TS   Dissolve 16.5 g of potassium iodide in water to 100 ml. This solution should be freshly prepared.

（5）Potassium iodobismuthate dilute TS   Dissolve 0.85 g of bismuth subnitrate in a mixture of 10 ml of glacial acetic acid and 40 ml of water. Before use, add 5 ml of potassium iodide solution （4→10）and 20 ml of glacial acetic acid to 5 ml of the solution mentioned above dilute with water to 100 ml.

（6）*p* – Dimethylaminobenzaldehyde TS   Dissolve 0.125 g of *p* – dimethylaminobenzaldehyde in a cooled mixture of 65 ml of nitrogen – free sulfuric acid and 35 ml of water, add 0. 05 ml of ferric chloride TS and mix well. This solution should be used within 7 days.

3. Carbohydrate

(1) Aniline – phthalate TS Dissolve 0. 93 g of aniline and 1. 66 g of o – phthalic acid in 100 ml of water saturated n – butanol. Different kinds of saccharide appear different colors. The detection of reducing sugar is more sensitive.

(2) α – Naphthol – sulphuric acid TS　Add 6. 5 ml of sulphuric acid slowly to 10. 5 ml of 15% alcoholic solution of α – Naphthol. Mix well and then add 40. 5 ml of alcohol and 4 ml of water. Mix well.

(3) Anisaldehyde – sulphuric acid TS　Dissolve 0. 5 ml of anisaldehyde of acetic acid, add 1 ml of sulphuric acid and mix well. This solution should be freshly prepared.

4. Phenolic compounds

(1) Diazobenzene sulfonic acid TS　Dissolve 1. 57 g of sulfonic acid in 80 ml of water and 10 ml of dilute hydrochloric acid under heating on a water bath. Cool to 15 ℃ and add 6. 5 ml of sodium nitrite solution (1→10) with stirring and dilute with water to 100 ml. This solution should be freshly prepared.

(2) Phloroglucinol – hydrochloric acid TS　Dissolve 0. 1 g phloroglucinol in ethanol to make 9 ml, and then dissolve 9 ml of hydrochloric acid, mix well. This solution should be freshly prepared.

(3) Iron chloride TS　Dissolve 9 g of iron chloride in water to make 100 ml. Phenols appear blue or green spot.

(4) Aluminum chloride TS　Dissolve 1 g of aluminum chloride in water to make 100 ml. It is used to detect flavone.

5. Quinone

Magnesim acetate TS　Dissolve 0. 5 g of magnesim acetate in methanol to make 100 ml. After puff, bake the spot for 5 minutes at 90 ℃. Then the quinone appears color.

6. Terpenoid

Vanillin – sulphuric acid TS　Dissolve 0. 1 g of vanillin in 10 ml of sulfuric acid. After puff bake the spot until it appears color.

7. Volatile oil

(1) Vanillin – sulphuric acid TS　Dissolve 0. 2 g of vanillin in 10 ml of sulfuric acid. After puff bake the spot until it appears color.

(2) Anisaldehyde – sulphuric acid TS　Dissolve 0. 5 ml of anisaldehyde in 50 ml of acetic acid, add 1 ml of sulphuric acid and mix well. This solution should be freshly prepared.

8. Steroid

Acetic anhydride – sulphuric acid TS　Dissolve 5 ml of acetic anhydride and 5 ml sulphuric acid, mix well in cooling condition, and then in dehydrated alcohol to make 50 ml. This solution should be freshly prepared. After puff bake the spot 10 for minutes. It is used to detect sterol and triterpenoid saponin.

9. Amino acids

Ninhydrin TS   Dissolve 2 g of ninhydrin in ethanol to make 100 ml.

10. Organic acid

（1）Bromphenol blue TS   Dissolve 0. 1 g of bromphenol blue in 3. 0 ml of sodium hydroxide solution（0. 05 mol/L）, and dilute with water to 200 ml.

（2）Bromocresol green TS   Dissolve 0. 04 g of bromocresol green in ethanol to make 100 ml. and then add sodium hydroxide solution（0. 1 mol/L）until appear blue color.

参 考 文 献

［1］吉丽娜，冯伟红，王智民，等．"一测多评"法与外标法测定三黄片中4种黄芩黄酮类成分［J］．中成药，2012，34（11）：2128－2133．

［2］杨菲，冯伟红，王智民，等．"一测多评"法测定银黄制剂中4种黄酮类成分含量［J］．中国药学杂志，2012，47（12）：87－92．

［3］Dandan Zhou，Yunhua Wang，Fan Li，etc. Study on HPLC fingerprint chromatography of Yiqifumai Injection. Chin J Pharm Anal，2009，9（11）：1900－1904．